The Well

Where Fitness Begins

From Within

Life Chronicles Publishing©2016

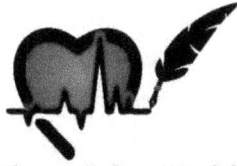

Life Chronicles Publishing
Give your life a voice!
mylifechronicles.org

ISBN-13: 9780692773024

ISBN-10: 0692773029

Cover Photo: Life Chronicles Publishing

Editor: Aisha Hollins

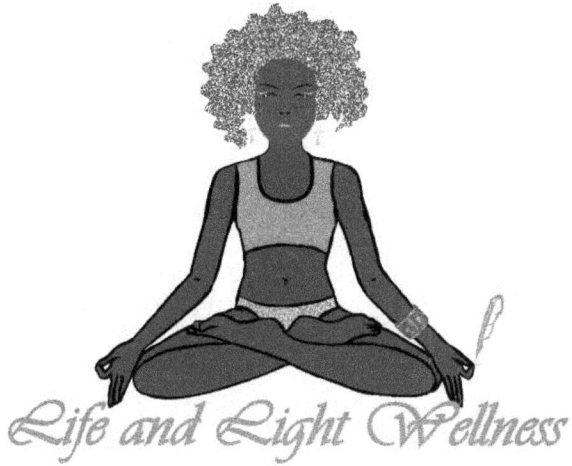

Life and Light Wellness

Life and Light Wellness, LLC.

Presents…

Table of Contents

Note To Readers

This book is an accumulation of experiences, ideas and opinions of the author, in addition to client testimonies and public data. The information in this book is intended to suggest to its readers an alternative path towards holistic transformation and heightened spiritual awareness.

All suggestions in this book should be examined thoroughly and any attempts at self-improvement based on opinions in this book should be consulted by the reader's physician or a competent professional prior to beginning a particular regimen. The information in this book is not intended to treat or diagnose any pre-existing conditions. The author, publisher and their affiliates make no promises or guarantees within the pages of this book and therefore waive all responsibility for any loss, personal and otherwise associated with the practices enclosed in this publication.

Dedication

To my tremendously supportive family and their various forms of loving support. To my husband, who was tired of seeing me miserable. His loving command to "Stop complaining and write," began a transformation within me that has continued to light my internal flame. I can't thank you enough for reminding me about the importance of personal accountability. To my mother, for her unwavering, consistent and transparent nurturing. Even when I've let fear take over, the confidence she's instilled in me always reigned supreme. To my father who showed me how to maneuver through this reality: It's to him I owe my diplomatic nature and financial savvy. Most importantly he showed me how a man should take care of his family. To my nephews, Anthony, Kai, and Sebastian who gave me a crash course in parenthood before I was blessed to deliver my own child. You all reminded me that the journey is to be embraced, not delayed. To my niece, Journee and "step" daughter Anya, thanks for reminding me to dance "just because" and the importance of girl time! And then there is Zoie, my Life and Light. If anything was ever worth the wait, it was you. I thank you for choosing me to usher you through this part of our journey. Your extreme self-awareness, confidence, innate intelligence, femininity and creativity give me life. You are "raising" me as much as I'm raising you and for that, I thank you. To my sister: our childhood antagonism has morphed into adult admiration. How far would we have gone without you honoring your journey and subsequently, me honoring mine? Thank you for showing the world that doing a 360 is absolutely possible. To my 4 sister-friends and 3 brother-friends. Not many people can say they're going 20+ years strong in a friendship. You all held me up in ways far too detailed to write. Let's keep our bond growing strong. To my step mom who always tells me, "You're going to be on Oprah's radar soon!" (hint, hint, O). To all my uncles, aunts and cousins: You never made me feel like I was alone. We are family in the truest sense of the word. To the Divine eye in I. Thank you for having you, me, and we, part of this master plan. I thank you for giving me all the MAGIC I need. To all my ancestors known and unknown: Because of you, I AM. Thank you for your everlasting imprint and support. This book is for all those reading it: for if it weren't for you saying, "Yes" to yourself, I wouldn't have received the message. Love all your lessons so you can learn to love your life.

WE ARE ONE

Part 1

Wisdom

I allow the lessons gained from all my experiences to plant seeds towards lifelong wisdom.

Sweeter than any dessert I've ever eaten, life is the sweetest, most deliciously rich treat I've tasted. In the closet lies my discovery. In the sun lies my energy. On my plate lies my therapy. On this journey lies my directory. In these words, lies our unity.

Foreword

Chop it up to being a child raised in the 80's. My mind was stimulated with images of Jane Fonda, Richard Simmons, Jack Lalane, Mr. T's physique, Carl Weather's swag, and my dad always working out. He was the epitome of strength: He was tall with lean muscle. He always found an opportunity to exercise. Early morning pushups (the memory of me hopping on his back while he did them…priceless), basketball and weekly baseball games, he did it all. He would even ride his bike to work sometimes just because. What stands out the most in my memory was that he ENJOYED it. He found intrinsic pleasure in exercise.

My mother: my beautiful, deep brown skinned mother with a perfect smile didn't enjoy exercise. I remember her and my aunt sweating away their unwanted weight by walking briskly in those silver "space suits" (more like bulky, insulated jogging suits). She was very conscious of her waistline (although as I child I never remember my mom being "big") and although she possessed all the feminine curves I imagine a woman would want, she was never completely happy with her look. Working out for my mom was strictly an extrinsic necessity.

I stayed active as a child. My mom bought me "Get In Shape, Girl"; the youth workout set that included a jump rope, headband, exercise mat and workout video. My sister would laugh at me as I got my sweat on…I was skinny as a rail. I wasn't body conscious at all back then. I was just a little girl who loved to be active. From jump rope-a-thons to running 1k's, from tetherball, kickball and dodge ball. I love it all!

As I hit my twenties I ran less and ate, partied and shopped more. This isn't to say I didn't enjoy an active lifestyle, however my fitness activities now took second place to my social activities. I didn't commit to a way of implementing them both equally, so the one that included more extrinsic value prevailed, and that was the nightlife. I never had a "weight" issue and I was a vegetarian for a few years at this time, so I rationalized in my twenty-something year old mind "party now, pay for it later." I haven't any regret for that mindset.

In my early to mid-thirties I grew tired of excessive partying, drinking and staying up late. Instinctively I knew a shift was coming. I started running again. I began to explore new areas to hike. I traveled to a lot of beach filled countries so I swam and snorkeled more. Fitness became more than working out, it was now a vehicle for discovery. This point in my journey reignited my passion for fitness and began my love for seeking wellness from an intrinsic standpoint.

When I used to hear the word fitness, I only associated it with how your body looked. I now know fitness is so much more. Fitness is defined as health. Health begins and ends internally. No amount of working out will do us any good if it not approached primarily from an internal perspective. Fitness begins from within.

The word *intrinsic* means something that's built in, genuine, something that is fundamentally yours. Discovery, enjoyment, fulfillment, peace and health are things that belong to us inherently. Intrinsic fitness and wellness have nothing to do with yo-yo diets, fads, or participating in anything excessively for the purpose of feeling high for a short amount of time. Intrinsic fitness is what we are born to experience, which is real health holistically: mind, spirit and body temple.

Approaching wellness from this perspective not only helped embrace a positive outlook toward health, it helped me attract a mate who loves exercise and is open to exploring deeper levels of what fitness is. This mindset also helped me possess the best health and body I've ever had, despite gaining sixty pounds while I was pregnant.

US indoors and outdoors champion hurdler Kellie Wells said, "If you tell yourself you're tired, or if you tell yourself you're sick, your body is going to follow your mind." Say to yourself that moving your body helps it flourish and you're mind agrees. Tell yourself that you despise fitness (health) for any reason, and your body will despise it. How you approach fitness and wellness determines your experiences within it. Working out and eating healthy can be viewed as a chore done only to maintain a look, or it can be approached as an opportunity to discover and implement exciting ways to attain and maintain health. Either way, the perception of it begins in the mind and this is what *The Well* will highlight: fitness of the mind and how to nurture your spirit and body temple.

I would have never thought at eight or nine years old that the influences of mom, dad, and "space suits", Carl Weathers, Jack Lalane, Mr. T and "Get In Shape, Girl" would've brought me here. But all our experiences are here to guide us to a place of purpose, not to a place of punishment. We are all here to change our thoughts, then change our behaviors, then finally change our lives, no matter what the driving force is in the moment. My mission is to open your mind to the very real possibility that you can and will obtain stellar wellness if you believe you can. Get to the root of your beliefs and you will enjoy the fruits of this amazing life.

`Infinite thanks for choosing me to guide you along this part of your journey and I thank you for seeking a better way for yourself. Besides, it's your right…intrinsically.

In Life and Light

Sahsha Campbell-Garbutt

Founder, Life and Light Wellness, LLC.

Chapter 1

Well-Come

You are exactly where you need to be.

Every thought, choice, and action you've made up to this moment has brought you here. You've arrived at a turning point; that roundabout in the road that you could've chosen to go right, left, or in a circle...right back to where you started. But you've made the responsible choice to go in another direction.

This direction, called responsibility, has lead you to a place where you're no longer satisfied with living a life less than spectacular. You've realized that you are not a spectator in your life, but an active participant. The activities you've engaged in prior to this point has brought you to the nosebleed seats in an arena as your life plays out on a stage in front of you. The power isn't in watching the play, feeling that you cannot change the script. The power lies in you going backstage and revamping the script. Consider this book the writers' studio. This is where you begin to revise your life.

The first thought you're probably having is "what's next"? You're asking, "How do I get from where I am, the nosebleed seats, to down there, backstage, without walking in the dark?" "The show has already begun. Is it fair for me to interrupt everyone's view by walking in front of him or her just so I can get backstage?" "What if I fall?" "What if I miss the show's climax while I'm trying to find my way?" Although those questions are valid, imagine your life is a Broadway play and in this show, you hold dual roles. You are the *producer;* (one with The Divine) you possess the ability to place, in this case, the proper thoughts and vibrations in line to manifest what you desire the most. You are also the *main character (*again, one with The Divine). With the proper *direction* (thoughts), you own and embrace your *role* (innate power). You determine how well the *play* (your life) is acted out. Your *performance* (the sum total of acknowledging, addressing, and transmuting your outdated thought patterns to manifest a fruitful life) determines how the *crowd* (people placed along your path to help make manifest your life's purpose) reacts to your play. Your performance determines if the crowd screams, *"encore"* (continuous help from The Universe to manifest your purpose) and it determines if other *opportunities* will present themselves, (reciprocity based on continual mental resetting) your *pay,* (receiving what you know your worth) and your ability to negotiate *higher wages* (the successful accomplishment of a task, which leads to greater confidence, greater manifestations and greater reward).

So, have no worry about whom you're going to interrupt as you make the necessary changes in your life. This book was written to interrupt expired and dysfunctional mindsets in order to guide you towards greater health and fitness. The key to successful health attainment, weight loss and subsequently, any personal goal(s), is to own the unhealthy mindsets and habits you have that are keeping your true desires from coming to fruition. Choosing to be responsible is the only way to make a change. You cannot change something you don't own up to, just as one cannot exchange items they've bought without having it in the first place.

Responsibility for the part you've played in an unfavorable position used to be taboo. We now understand that responsibility is the key that unlocks the door to the house of health and happiness. You can hardly experience one fully without being in possession of the other (although even those with dis-ease can choose to be happy which can potentially jump start the healing process). So, while some continue with shortcuts in an effort to avoid getting uncomfortable with past and present choices, you've now chosen to custom-pave the long road because it's down this path that you'll gain all the experience you need for long lasting success. Taking shorts is your declaration to The Divine and yourself that you're not worth the time it takes for cultivating greatness. Shortcuts translate that you're satisfied with short-lived success, short-term happiness, short-term relationships and short-term weight loss. NOTHING LONG LASTING WILL BE CREATED WITH SHORT CUTS.

Most weight is regained that was removed via liposuction not because the procedure failed, but because the procedure didn't teach the person to develop the new habits needed for maintaining a healthy body weight. Most weight is regained once you stop eating packaged diet food because while eating what's in the bag, there was little understanding of what to eat outside of it. There's one thing to be told what to do, but there's a

9

whole world to be gained by participating in what you must do to reach where you want to be. Protecting your child from harm is one thing, but preventing your child from learning the lessons he or she needs to arm them in survive life's "rough patches" can be detrimental. Preventing yourself from adopting new mindsets that translate into new habits can leave you hopping from diet to diet, and detour to detour.

The long road doesn't have to be hard. The road is equipped with a variety of circumstances specifically designed to ensure your successful and enjoyable journey. Your navigation (Divine Center) WILL NOT fail you. The only thing that can fluctuate is your ability to listen and even that can be fixed…if you choose to recognize without guilt or shame that it's in need of repair.

The road to wellness is just like being in any learning institution. Just as the first day of school brings anticipation and excitement, so will this. As you become acclimated with the course and its teachings and what it takes to succeed, you become adaptable and receptive to the revelations that come with it. And just like during test time, nervousness will set in, but once you trust that within you lies what it takes to pass the test; what it takes to live in control of what goes into your mind and your mouth, you pass it or in this case you gain the readiness to receive "promotion". You're ready for more: mind, spirit, and body temple.

So, continue to let the momentum of your choice to go in another direction guide you to the mind and body you deserve. May you anticipate long lasting weight release as long as you're releasing the mental, emotional and physical baggage obtained from lack of knowledge. The stage is set for your success. Internal lights and camera are on. Now, it's time for some action.

Chapter 2

The Well-Thin Detox

While on day three of my most recent full body detox, I was watching a documentary on the sugar industry and the effects it has on the mind and body. A mentor of mine said she was home watching a documentary on sugar that Friday night, so I figured I'd do the same on a Saturday night with my daughter. A man in the film, who was obese and admittedly addicted to soft drinks, described what he was going through as he allowed his body to become sugar-free. As I watched it: lethargic, fatigued and a little on edge, I realized that Sahsha, Intrinsic Wellness Guide and Plant-Based Advocate was having sugar withdrawals. The greater realization I had was not only those obsessed with sugar, but those also hooked on salt, drugs (albeit legal or not), shopping, gambling, sex, alcohol, tobacco, stress, drama, or fear can ONLY go through withdrawals if addicted. I was addicted to sugar.

What does addiction look like? Take me for example. At 39 I'm toned, happy, and always have something positive to say. I eat a lot of greens, drink homemade smoothies, meditate and stay active. I have a loving husband, great kids and supportive family and friends. My business is growing at lightning speed and I'm thrilled to be living in the greatest times that have ever existed. Yet, I've always been comforted by refined sugar. I don't drink Starbucks on a regular basis and you won't see me eating donuts, a lot of bread, drinking alcohol, or fruit juice, but I sure do love my cookies, cakes, and brownies. I had my moments that I would eat a piece of chocolate a day, every day...occasionally with a cookie or brownie to accompany it. Since the aforementioned was intact, I DESERVED a treat... Okay, an indulgence...almost daily. "Sugar doesn't kill anyone... really" is what I spoke to myself. Truth is, ANYTHING in excess is one of two things: a lethal weapon OR a distraction from what's keeping you from becoming a lethal weapon. In my moment of detox: no meat, dairy, refined sugar, starch, nothing processed or heavily cooked, I was somewhat forced to face that which I've allowed myself to be distracted from: the why. Why, in my case, can I either minimize or completely let go of white rice, pasta, dairy, meat, hard alcohol, eggs, but not refined sugar? What does this chemical do to me that I cannot bring forth within myself? Where did this all start? When did it go from a pleasure to a habit, to a full-on addiction? I was like a junkie on a corner looking for her next fix. Sugar went from a recreational thing to a down right necessity. And similar to a junkie, I would have streaks of "being clean" to streaks of "binging mean". It had its root, and I was hell bent on digging it up. This time wasn't the time before. It was now, and my mind was made up. I will conquer this addiction.

The things I thought I easily reduced weren't reduced at all. It was replaced with my overconsumption of desserts. White rice and other processed foods had the same effect on me as the brownie itself. Research led me to understand that the processing of certain foods stripped it of almost all its nutritive value only leaving behind a sugary residue that I was consuming in droves. This kept me going under the guise that I was reducing my sugar intake. Unbeknownst to me, I was

13

replacing one form of sugar with its healthier looking, heavily promoted counterpart, starch. No rehab facility would knowingly give one addicted to meth, cocaine instead if the goal is to truly heal them, so why would the food industry offer the consumer highly addictive sugary foods under the assumption that its better than the desserts they were consuming before? Maybe it's because the food industry's job isn't to make us healthier but to keep their pockets heftier. No matter the reasoning, it became clear to me that processed sugar is strategically placed in, or is created from, the act of processing food. The only chance I had to allow this addiction to subside was to break away from my consumption of packaged foods altogether, or at least until I was mentally strong enough to eat it responsibly on occasion.

Twenty Days without what???

The particular detox I completed took no shorts and, why should it? Short cuts never lead to long-term successes and the one thing I wanted to experience…finally, was infinite freedom from in my case, sugar. If I could relinquish the need for a substance that was keeping me from optimal living, what more could I accomplish? What other shortcomings could I overcome if I addressed and abolished this block? Admitting what I was addicted to without shame was the first step in regaining the quality of life I NEEDED to have, in order to live the life, I believed I was truly intended to live; one full of vigor, vitality, and voraciousness. Allowing myself to blame society, the food industry, my family or any other social circumstance was only going to prevent me from successfully conquering sugar. Circumstances are an opportunity to correct misinformation. It's The Divine's way of lending us experiences

14

to expand our existence while on this plane. My intent was to first conquer sugar, then the other parts of myself that weren't properly aligned.

The 20 days I went without comfort foods, I was able to discover things about myself that I was previously unaware of. I discovered that just because I love hot food doesn't mean that all my food has to be cold. A lot of fruits and vegetables last longer unrefrigerated, so enjoying raw, room temperature foods is something I did then, and I still practice now. Getting creative with food preparation and watching others enjoy the fruits of my food "deprivation" helped me to discover the myriad of foods there are to appreciate without added sugars or heat, and it opened up others to the possibility of not only eating clean but enjoying the taste and nutritional value of real food.

Even though I thought I ate pretty healthy before, I enjoyed my food overly seasoned and overly cooked which prevented me from discovering the true flavor and uniqueness of the fruits and vegetables I consumed. In changing my diet, I now see that I was trying to DUPLICATE the tastes of the meats and starches I previously ate as opposed to APPRECIATING the whole foods for its distinctive flavors. I was subconsciously sabotaging my success by holding on to my past food experiences believing it was the best food experiences. Did I want to overcome the attachment to meat and cheese by making my food taste cheesy and meaty? That's not the way. Although there's nothing wrong with enjoying what you like, don't force your new way of eating and living to mimic your past. In essence, by being open to enjoying a new thing for what it IS allows the chance to change what was experienced BEFORE. The biggest lesson for me in all of this was to enjoy the present because it's new and to anticipate the future because it's a chance to renew. Success is experienced in the NOW, in THIS PRESENT MOMENT when you say YES to the unknown. Begin to wrap your mind around that.

Prior to this particular detox, this very book in your possession was laid into my lap while meditating. Soon after I received this as a Divine Message, people began asking me if I had an online or written fitness program, as if they were confirming what I was given from within. It was cool indeed. But with any big idea comes big responsibility and with that comes big change. I knew I wasn't exempt from that rule. Let the self-excavating begin.

I couldn't shake the feeling of how this project was going to be THAT thing: that ONE thing that catapulted people from wanting to get free to actually walking in their freedom. But as I couldn't release that feeling, I also felt a burden on me, like a thick smoke had replaced the oxygen I breathed. I felt like I was carrying a vibrational load that could no longer be supported by my current state of being: doubtful, unmindful and riddled with excuses. My responsibility to write a book to help people recalibrate their thoughts and as a byproduct, attain their weight loss goals or any life goals, was only going to work if I recalibrate my thoughts which would set me free from my sugar dependency. The only way to do that was to confront the mindset that got me there in the first place.

For me, and all of you reading this, to spring into action, I had to go into my "dark closet" and do some spring-cleaning.

Those perceived as healthy and fit, or those wealthy as sh!t, are revered as successful based on appearances. But when perception isn't enough for those "living the dream", what happens next? For some, the illusion leads them into a whirlwind of excessive living, recklessness, and depression. For those no longer supported by their self-made façade, the journey takes them towards a path of introspection. The word itself implies that the route taken will lead one to inspect them self from an internal aspect: your thoughts, opinions, beliefs, characteristics, and experiences, to see how they've served you, where they currently have you, and, will they take you to where you want to be.

Going into "the dark", until recently, wasn't something encouraged by pop culture. Why bring up things that can stir up old, uncomfortable feelings, when you can simply take a pill or eat a meal to feel better if even for a moment? Those habits have led to an overly depressed, overtly violent, extremely overworked and increasingly obese population who has been conditioned to deflect their challenges and ignore their "gut" cry for freedom. The same feeling that leads us to say, in hindsight "I should have trusted my gut!" is being silenced in shame, medication, and toxic overload. When wealth, religion, status, manmade substances or Internet sensationalism can no longer quell the nudge from within to "come holla at me", we must take heed. We must pause.

The most beautiful things are made in the dark: it's where diamonds gain their durability and brilliance, it's where life is conceived, grown, and prepared for delivery, and it's where your body rests while it's being tuned up for the day ahead. It's also where you go to emerge free from past experiences, systematic traumas, and stale mindsets. Why avoid the beauty of darkness?

The relationship you build with yourself tends to work best when you can be honest about your feelings and current desires. Honesty brings simplicity of choice because when you recognize, love and accept who you are in the PRESENT, when you allow yourself to step away from your PAST identity (most likely given to you from an environment who never discovered themselves) and when you grant yourself permission to live in a space of gratitude and expectancy towards the FUTURE, your choices become simple and you'll begin to move in a direction that serve your highest good. In making choices I now ask myself this simple question. "Will doing what's presented to me lead me towards my mission?" If it does, I move. If it doesn't, I walk away. There's power and peace that comes from making life simple, but that can only be activated when we engage in some "alone time" with ourselves. You will be hard pressed to improve any area of your life based on things you don't recognize as internal roadblocks. There's a lot of health to gain from a physical detox but there's even more emotional wealth to be discovered once you free those "skeletons" in your mental closet.

Chapter 3

Take It Out The Closet: How To Recognize, Release, & Redesign Outdated Mental Blocks

I used to watch the show *Hoarders* in disgust. I couldn't quite wrap my head around their reality. How could they feel so comfortable, so attached to all that... junk? How could they continually make excuses for holding on to old pieces of trash, expired food, and non-functional appliances? The hoarders fought tooth and nail to justify themselves dwelling in filth, mainly because they knew that any other rationale would mean letting go of their mess and reshaping their lives. They don't realize that *letting go* simply means claiming ownership of what they created so it can be released while making space for something new. Instead, most chose to keep a tight grip on their painful past as an excuse to hoard. It provided comfort to them because they still held on to the moments where they felt lost or abandoned, or perhaps, they held on to those objects because those things represented a time where they felt completely in control. Whichever the case, hoarding creates an illusion of reign over their environment because they believe OTHERS have control of how they feel, which is why the participants on that show became extremely defensive when others tried to help them release their clutter.

Hoarders hold on to so much, they forget just how much they're holding on to! Ignoring your surroundings, internally and externally, will do that. They don't realize that the objects they covet are nothing more than pain made tangible. Without it they think they're no one. If the items are trashed, what excuse exists for them to live a life in fear?

They sense responsibility knocking at their door, and that odor is enough to keep the closet door shut. They begin to see that responsibility is the light switch that needs to be turned on in order to truly live. The light of responsibility gives us the faith needed to trust our experiences as moments of promotion, not persecution. Claiming responsibility for the choices previously made is where freedom lies. Why? Because when one chooses to see their missteps, they are less likely to stumble over the same thing twice! It's hard to avoid things not acknowledged, right? You become free to move forward because you no longer fear the mistake behind you! You simply choose to understand how the experience was supposed to benefit you. But the reality is, freedom and choice are terrifying options if you've never used them. Although they're the birthright of all humans, the belief that one can be free from any aspect of their past can be paralyzing, like riding a bike without the support of training wheels. Walking in a space where you no longer make excuses for your current condition means knowing you have a greater purpose despite of your previous experiences. Most define themselves by what happened to them, not WHY it happened to them, and WHAT they're to take from the experience. Once you truly believe that all pain is to facilitate growth, your perspective shifts from powerlessness to powerful. Your perception morphs from "woe is me" to "wow, look at me" outwit, outshine and outsmart any obstacle!

When the day of reckoning arrives, anxieties and doubts kick in, as the hoarders have to confront all their junk. They begin to feel it's easier to keep it all in the closet that to expose it for a moment and subsequently, be free for a lifetime.

With great hesitation, they start sorting through their piles of mess and their emotions get shaken up. They begin to see things they thought were forgotten; an old picture stirs up memories of a past relationship. Reading a fifty-year-old letter reignites the passion they once had about fulfilling a dream, as they begin to ask themselves again why they abandoned their dream in the first place. Sorting through their mess isn't easy, but most of them, realizing that those who support them see no abashment in their process, continue to sort through AND now separate things into two piles: what serves them, and what doesn't. Once the process is done, not only has their physical environment been transformed, but they too, look as if they've had a makeover, and indeed they have. Years have been taken off their faces and bodies because they have released the years of perceived torment from their minds. They have turned what they used to believe was a tragedy into triumph by simply examining and transmuting their physical and mental surroundings. Cleaning the junk out of their homes was made possible for them by their own willingness to research the various experiences they've encountered, now understanding that those things happened for them to grow. Because of their newfound belief, they're now able to create a happy space for those experiences to not only be transmuted but also celebrated within them. They are now renewed because they realize they are not a product of their experiences, but a by-product of the lessons learned from it!

Does any of this sound familiar? Of course, you don't believe that those exclusively featured on *Hoarders* are the only ones who hold on to a lot of "things" as a way to cover up their underlying pain, right? We at some point, are, or used to be hoarders of past thoughts, old experiences, and non-functional reasoning that has kept our misinterpreted emotions in a dark closet. We either have, or are still choosing to bury fear under the blanket, in an effort to not revisit the pain, not realizing that when its hidden is when it's hurting the most. Bringing light to a past that's holding us hostage in the present is like acknowledging a physical pain in order for it to receive the treatment needed for better mobility. The time is now to bring light to what has been clouded in darkness.

My closet was a mess. I buried the shame of never completing my degree, losing my home, abandoning various romantic relationships because "the thrill was gone", aborting a child and not sticking with previous business ventures under my superwoman suit and sugar consumption. That suit no longer fit though, and I was FORCED to LOSE the WEIGHT of the masquerade. My issue was abandonment, and I declared that once I got it out the closet, it was never going to occupy that space again.

"Sahsha, Why didn't you complete your degree?" asked self. Wait; did you think this was some formal ritual you had to go through with the help of some external intercessor? The process of realigning your mental space is as simple and raw as asking yourself the questions that have ALWAYS lingered in your mind.

"I didn't complete my degree because I was bored in school and had a lot going on in my personal life." "What did the things you had going on

22

in your life have to do with you while you were in class? You were making great grades, so why stop attending school?" said self. "I was thinking of home life and what I didn't have more than my school life and all the other things I did have at my disposal. I chose to let my thoughts be somewhere that wasn't going to help me leave the very situation that had me distracted", said Sahsha. "Oh, I see. It seems to me that just as you were reaching your peak at school and you felt the pressure during finals week, you chose to deal with a more familiar pressure, that being your home life, while abandoning your eminent scholastic success. School was going too easy, and since you were taught that success couldn't be easy, and although you weren't sure of the direction you wanted to go in your education and yes, you wanted to pursue modeling, the two you chose to pursue was entertainment and familiar instinct instead of entertainment and education. You did great in modeling, but when it appeared you reached your plateau, you blamed yourself for not having anything solid to fall back on. As opposed to owning the choice you made in that moment, you blamed your circumstances for your choices instead of your choice for your circumstance. You went in search of another degree without researching the degree to which you've learned your lesson: Abandonment is aborting the commitment to yourself, NOT your circumstances. No matter what you think your running from, that very thing stays alive in your mind until you see it for what it is, and more importantly, for what it's there to provide you. You now know that you're here for more than what a formal education and entertainment can ever afford you. The loss and abandonment you chose was for you to GAIN a sense of your true purpose. Your overconsumption of sugar was because you were chasing the feeling; that sweet spot you felt you couldn't get from your life. You, and the fulfillment of your purpose IS the high of life you are seeking. You understand that now, right? "Affirmed self. My card was pulled. And I, in shock of what I'd suppressed under the shelter of an ultra-fit body filled with sugary foods, kick-ass writing skills, and the ability to help others progress, replied with a major exhale... "Yes." And then, the tears came to wash away any remaining maybes.

Just as cleaning out our physical closet is done a few times a year, the process of cleaning out our mental closets should be, and for me, is done on a regular basis. For every summit that is climbed, we all must walk down the mountain. The difference is now I walk with my head high and my eyes fixed; not on the next summit, but on the road ahead that will lead me there. I now enjoy life's peaks AND valleys.

What does all this have to do with fitness, you ask? This has EVERYTHING to do with fitness! Long lasting fitness cannot be attained unless you retrain your mind to curve the emotional responses it has towards food. Your mind is the dashboard for your body's emotional responses. The mind is similar to a muscle. If you don't strengthen it with expansive thoughts and rejuvenating foods, it will atrophy, like any unused muscle. With kind, loving attention to your thoughts surrounding WHY you desire the food you do and WHAT triggers those cravings, you can get to the root of your emotions and begin to accept a new food reality! The endorphins released from sugar consumption is what you crave, regardless of the source, so the sweetness of an apple can be just as enjoyable as the sweetness of a cookie, with a lot more nutritional value, if you tell your mind so. The reality is simple; we are ORGANIC beings. We are ONE with the nature that surrounds us. The food we were meant to enjoy, the foods made specifically for our expansion come from an ORGANIC source, our earth. If the majority of our food consumption comes from an INORGANIC (factory made) source, we will suffer. Period. Once that belief becomes your unchangeable reality, you will never have to diet again. Diets only come into place when you consume MORE factory-made foods than those that are "manufactured" from The Divine Source. You deserve a higher quality of life; therefore, from life you should eat. When your mind believes that, your body WILL respond with vitality and as a result, a strengthened mind, weight loss, refined health, higher energy, and much more! The weight you desire to lose is just as much emotional as it is physical, and I truly believe that approaching fitness from the inside out is the only true way to release it.

I am a product of the beauty within the dark closet. I am continuously healing, transmuting and growing because I refuse to be a victim of mindsets that no longer serve me, ideologies that were never meant for me, and systems that don't expand me. I am anti-ignorance and pro transmutation. I'm an advocate for getting to the root of things. I am fed up with institutions whose primary agenda is to keep you in a state of stalled out growth for monetary gains. There is an alternative, and the alternative is you. And that alternative begins in the mind for as your mind speaks, your body responds in action.

The word *guide* means "to assist one or to reach a destination in, an unfamiliar area by giving direction..." This book includes a series of exercises you will perform on yourself to *guide* you to a place of self-love and self-value. This book also includes affirmations to replace the words you previously used to describe yourself: words that didn't come from a place of acceptance and understanding. Also included are meditation, detoxification, nutrition, and exercise suggestions that will help you not only achieve your fitness goals, but also if practiced, will lead you towards fulfilling your life goals.

I feel you've now accepted how exciting the process of change can be. You accept the responsibility that comes with change is nothing more than premium gas needed to fuel the high-end vehicle that is you. Your vehicle requires certain maintenance to function as it was made to. The maintenance we all require, called responsibility, addresses the need for mental and physical tunes ups as well as knowing when we are in overdrive and when we require rest. Responsibility, just like car maintenance, entails getting our exterior detailed as well. But just as one wouldn't spend thousands of dollars refurbishing the exterior of a car whose engine isn't working, why would you spend an immeasurable amount of time in the gym, buying diet food, at the salon, or even eating clean, without addressing any weaknesses of the heart and mind, which are the key components that keep your engine running? Running away from self-responsibility doesn't erase it, but walking through it with a sound mind can change how you see it. Just as a car breaks down and can be fixed, so can you. Even when you stumble along this journey, you can choose to get back up. But you can no longer avoid or deflect responsibility, if you want to move through your past into your present.

It's your responsibility to choose to make moves that will propel you, and propulsion will NEVER take you backward.

    I'm no doctor, guru or expert. I'm a lady who chose to get to the root of my lessons so I could plant new seeds in my mind. I'm a woman who sees that no matter how much material things we've been afforded in this life, it's the quality of how we view our life experiences that determines how much we can truly enjoy them. I am my own experiment. I know it's no one's job to know me better than me and if I relinquish that right, I will continue to be a victim to the protocols and ideologies of others. And more so, I'm a mother, wife, daughter, sister, aunt, niece, cousin, friend, plant based advocate, intrinsic wellness coach, fitness fan, writer, author, new reality creator, music and sunshine lover who KNOWS she's here to help people rediscover their inner light so they can stop going in circles trying to chase a light outside of them. Within us all lays *The Well* that once replenished, can sustain us along this wonderful journey called life. You're tired of yo-yo diets and up and down emotions. Let's put an end to that…together. Weight loss can be attained if you choose to release your emotional pain. The only time to start is NOW. You are MORE than well equipped.

Part 2

WORDS

The words I heard were the storm,

The words I hear are the seeds,

The words I speak are the rain,

They now have permission to wash away all my pain.

Chapter 4

Why a Wellness Protract?

There's a power in words; and when you sign the dotted line on your intentions, you now own it and the commitment to its fulfillment. Contracts hold businesses and consumers liable for not adhering to its terms; This PROTRACT (pro meaning "for" and tract meaning "an expanse of area or land) on the other hand, is to support the expansion of your mind, faith, and territory both physically and spiritually. Once one goal is achieved a spark is lit, and the desire to achieve greater things is ignited. The belief in your innate power goes from invisible to invincible as the fruits of your labor make manifest right before your eyes.

It is completely normal to feel fear or doubt. This is a new thing and with all new things comes a sense of hesitation. What you're feeling is nothing more than an overactive imagination attempting to paint a picture of an experience that's yet to happen. To avoid anxiety, just enjoy each moment for what it is; a step in a new direction. As your paintbrush gets dampened so to speak, the picture you paint will represent a reinvigorated, not reminiscent version of you.

Trust your past as it's prepared you for your present. Trust your present as it's filled with purpose. Trust your path as it's led you here, to the place where you say YES to a new mind, a new body and a renewed life!

Why Weight?

"Now I will take the load from your shoulders; I will free your hands from their heavy tasks" – Psalm 81:6 (NLT)

You'd be hard pressed not to notice the vast amount of changes occurring in our world. Times, we all believed were behind us are reappearing with tremendous force. The only things that have the ability to resurface themselves are the things that were never completely resolved. Societal imbalances of every kind are resurrecting because laws were set up to placate them, not eradicate them. Relationships that seem to have ended decades ago are reemerging not because of loneliness or lack of options, but because of lessons missed or perhaps, love regained. The same too, can be said for those who deal with weight "issues". The issue is reoccurring not only because they've ignored their unsatisfactory diet and exercise habits, but also because they haven't "let go" of unnecessary emotional weight.

What are you holding on to?

Most with weight challenges have dealt with them more than once in their lives. The constant spinning of the weight loss wheel is a tiring task that can leave you with more questions than answers. For those of you reading this who's facing body weight challenges, or any reoccurring challenges for that matter, answering this one question can unlock the door to lightweight living: what are you carrying?

Are you holding on to age-old disappointment from a failed venture? Are you attached to the guilt associated with staying in an unhealthy relationship? Perhaps you are STILL blaming yourself for not passing the BAR or CBEST?

Imagine if you would, all that emotional weight in a heavy basket affixed to your right shoulder with your left and right hands keeping it steady. The way you walk…the way you live your life is dependent upon keeping the basket on your shoulder. You walk with apprehension so the basket doesn't fall. Your hands are constantly carrying your burdens so you have no room to invite the opportunity to shake someone's hand, touch soft fabric or embrace something new. You've made no space to invite new results because your hands are tied to things of old. Have you ever stopped to imagine how much simpler life would be and how much lighter your journey could be if you emptied the basket and took it off your shoulders?

In order to effectively and permanently release the weight that's plagued your physical body, you must be willing to let go of your emotional load. The correlation isn't commonly made between those who have released weight and kept it off versus those who constantly ride the weight exchange rollercoaster, but I'd like to challenge you to consider that if you're doing everything "right"; eating clean and exercising, and the weight is still sticking around there's a possibility that what your carrying is a load of emotionally energy that is preventing you from experiencing physical freedom.

It is not your responsibility to carry mistakes. The only responsibility you have is to learn the lessons from your experiences. Carrying an emotional load translates to your physical body that you are not ready or willing to release the baggage, and therefore the weight, of yesterday; you have not learned the lesson.

School is back in session. Declare that this moment is the moment you will past the test that has been plaguing you for lifetimes. Forgive yourself. You're just a student of life. Drop the emotional weight and invite a space of weightlessness to invade your mind and body temple. The burden was a blessing in disguise, an asset to your journey. So, go ahead; free up your hands, put the basket down and embrace the possibility of a new life and body with arms wide open. Why weight?

The Wellness Protract

I, _____ am The Well. Within me dwells an inherent abundance of what is needed to achieve self-defined success. Inside lies a personal definition of perfection, purpose, and passion that will always allow the waters of life to flow in me and through me. I give myself permission to keep my well full by partaking in activities that nourish and replenish my entire being. I am one with The Divine Source and because of that, I have direct access to what I need, when I need it. As knowledge is gained and wisdom is applied, I use it to free my mind and release my body of all things toxic and replace it with sustaining thoughts, actions, and foods. As my thoughts become realigned, my body will follow. From here on out, I'll only walk down the path that leads me towards the infinite waters that are my Well. And if I go astray, I give myself permission to continue where I left off. I am The Well, and all is well.

Signature _____

Date _____

Chapter 5

The Water: 30 Motivations To Replenish Your Well

No matter what walk of life you're from or how far you are on your amazing journey, you can use some motivation along the way. But for those who are walking along a new path, an added dose of motivation can help ensure success in reaching your destination!

For so many years, you've been filled up with words that have now become your belief, words that do not give your life or proper perspective of who you are and your capability. Those same words must be swapped out with verbiage that will REPLACE past mindsets. It's a challenge to attain weight release if you keep saying, "I'm so fat" and it will be tough to attract a life mate if you keep repeating, "I'm so unlucky in love". Whatever your desires are, they come to fruition from what you BELIEVE, which translates into what you SPEAK. Words are powerful indeed, and since the intention of this book is for you to understand that you possess the POWER to create the reality you wish, the following thirty motivations were written with your power in mind!

Read them daily, multiple times a day. As weird as you may think it sounds to assert them aloud, do it! I truly accept that words carry vibrations and when spoken from love, they resonate with the love space within our core. You have NOTHING to lose but negative self-talk…and a little body weight as a result!

The Water…

The words I speak are the WATER that quenches my thirst for positive reinforcement.

The only choices I choose to make are those that will lead me down my chosen path. If I stray, I give myself permission to begin again, knowing my path always welcomes me.

I will no longer interfere with my body's natural desire to heal.

What I want in the physical has already manifested, and I allow my mind to catch up to it.

I am willing to go three weeks without the things that keep me in my comfort zone knowing that long-term comfort only leads to complacency.

I DESERVE MORE THAN I'M USED TO!

I am a willing participant in the rejuvenation of my mind and body.

Responsibility is the end of recess and the beginning of your marathon. Consistency and clarity WILL win the race.

MY END GOAL BEGINS NOW!

I am one with nature. I no longer resist the natural process of change.

Waiting to accomplish a task, without any set action plan, is waiting for a time that will never exist. Action = Results!

Others understanding your life aren't prerequisites for you to live yours.

Perfection began at inception. I've been deemed excellent from birth. What I'm striving for isn't perfection, but a recollection of all my worth.

I have NOTHING to lose but my old way of thinking, feeling, looking and eating!

I AM THE ANSWER I'VE BEEN LOOKING FOR!

I only desire the foods that help me thrive, strive, and come alive!

I'm no longer DISabled in my INability to accept REsponsibility for my past. I now know my UNlimited power lies in my PREdestined future!

The body I had was to support my tests. The body I will have is to support my testimonies.

I am a Divine flower honored for its beauty. I give thanks for the processes involved that have lead me to this present moment.

I regret nothing. I reflect on everything. I expect greatness.

I love the foods that fuel my body, strengthen my heart, and nourish my soul.

My body is a magnificent vehicle made with its own lane and I'll stay in it. My lane has no room for comparison or criticism.

I was born to experience success. NOTHING can change that.

Attaining good health isn't a passing phase, but a constant stage in my life.

I love myself and because of that love, I'm willing to apply what's best for me on a daily basis.

If what I eat is made in a plant, I will remain on a mental plantation. IF what I eat IS the plant, like a plant, I will grow.

I thank the PAST for showing me what I no longer want. I celebrate the PRESENT for showing me what I need in order to have the FUTURE I deserve!

My body IS my temple, no matter what size it is.

Releasing the heaviness of the past opens the door to experience a light-filled future.

Fitness is: <u>F</u>inally <u>I</u>ntending <u>T</u>o <u>N</u>ail <u>E</u>xperiences of <u>S</u>weet <u>S</u>uccess

My words will not return void. My intentions are set. My will IS done, and I am thankful!

Chapter 6

Let's Get Accountable:

...Because there's no one accountable for you, but you.

Habits aren't broken overnight. Even after a decision is made, there's always going to be a level of hesitancy in taking the first step onto the bridge of change. Part of the uncertainty lies in the question: "Where do I begin?" The reality of changing a lifetime of habits can appear daunting to say the least, but once you develop within yourself your own way of establishing methods of change, you will begin to feel in control of all aspects of your life. This isn't to say that the methods others use don't work, but since most people are attempting to break the chains of how others taught them to think, live, and speak, it's important to formulate an approach to living that doesn't negate your unique experiences and desires. Once you trust yourself enough to see that you inherently know what's best for you, there's nothing wrong with taking bits and pieces from the plans of those who've successfully defined happiness for themselves! You've spent a lifetime working towards, and aiding in, the manifestation of the dreams and wishes of others, but now is the time to put the work in to remodel your temple the exact way you see it fit!

So why have I written this book as a guide if I'm encouraging you to honor your own path? For the same reason an athlete has a trainer in addition to his or her natural ability, or like a child who uses training wheels until he or she is comfortable without them, this book is a support manual, followed by your God given intelligence, to aid in your transition from a life conditioned to a life filled with unconditional love and freedom. The need to please others despite how the aftermath may affect you mustn't trump your own well-being. That habit fosters the fear of not being accepted by others, and the acceptance of others will never satisfy you long term. The first step towards a fit body is recognizing the mindsets that have prevented you from a fit mind. These exercises are meant to jog your memory and flex your perception of the experiences you had, but were never able to embrace.

Feed Your Mind (the good stuff) And The Rest Will Follow

As someone who's worked as a personal trainer and as a fitness lover, the one thing everyone wants to do is get fit fast! "Sahsha, what is the best exercise to do to tone up my body?" My typical reply was, "any series of movements that utilize your biggest muscles like your quads." My new response: Your mind.

Although your mind is not really a muscle, it works like one. Whatever you feed it, whether positively or negatively, multiplies. Whatever belief systems and interpretations of your experiences that are embedded in your internal garden called the subconscious navigates your thoughts;

your thoughts feed your mind, and whatever triggers it determines what you eat and subsequently what your body and life look like.

So, all the time spent utilizing physical activity to release weight could have been potentially split in half if we had simply focused on our subconscious beliefs and our emotional triggers, which to a huge degree determine what we desire to eat? YES.

You Can't Hurry Up, Cuz You've Got Too Much Stuff

The line above is an excerpt from soul singer Erykah Badu's hit song, "Bag Lady." She hit the nail on the head when she sang about holding on to emotional dead weight as if it were heavy baggage. Throughout the song, she spoke of, in essence, missed opportunities and physical pain that manifest if emotional baggage isn't released. The bags cannot be seen, but can be felt by those who are carrying it and by those who are in the presence of the carrier. In any case, it serves no benefit. The song is art, imitating life.

Most of us are carrying an emotional weight and an energetic load so heavy that it delays progression in every area of our life. What makes this weight so difficult to release is that it's not always visible to our two eyes, yet it's felt to our core. And in a world where we barely have the time to breath, let alone feel ourselves, it comes as no surprise that we ignore our ill feelings until we can no longer hide their damaging effects. We must FIRST begin to release the weight in our hearts caused by guilt, pain, jealousy, and regret before we can release the weight in our bodies *We've been focusing on releasing the wrong weight.*

Close your eyes and visualize carrying emotional weight as the equivalent to hauling physical baggage. Each unresolved, misunderstood and misinterpreted experience that isn't utilized as energetic fuel (progressive energy) is packed away, much like how an excess of unprocessed protein and carbs is stored as sugar and fat. If our emotional state "tips the scales", they have the opportunity to add extra weight to our energy fields…meaning the space within us that occupies our dreams, desires, and believes etc. If dead weight is occupying our energy space, there will be no room to receive that which you are calling into your life. **The energy in you is the energy around you.** Under those circumstances, there is no room to lose weight; there is only room to lose hope. But that's not what we are hear for, is it. We are here for WHOLE-istic fitness. This is where the bags get released.

What Is A Fit Mind?

When most people hear the word *fitness,* they automatically think of strenuous exercise and that's understandable. Our conditioning has lead us to believe that in order to be fit we must be muscle clad or have the body fat percentage of a teenager, and neither of those are true. Fitness is simply defined as health and health is primarily internal. Putting an emphasis on our subconscious, emotional and mental fitness is paramount, yet it's the missing component in most of our lives. And since our mental fitness determines how well we navigate along this adventure called life, I feel this is the perfect time to develop the attributes needed to strengthen the most powerful tool we have called the mind. *A fit mind is a healthy mind whose thoughts have the power to redefine the past, revitalize the present, and redesign the future from one that would create despair to one that creates a destiny, which brings forth happiness and fulfillment.*

The Attributes Of A Fit Mind

Just as you would take steps or develop a formula with your physical body to get it looking the way you envision, there are certain characteristics needed to develop a fit mind. Below outlines the 5-step process needed to develop a fit mind.

Appraisal: Examine your thoughts and where it has brought you thus far. Look with a loving eye at how you interpret all your previous experiences and trace the roots of your beliefs without judgment. Judgment is a heavy weight to carry.

Acceptance: Embrace the current space you're in. Learn from it. It's nothing more or less than a reflection. The MORE you accept that your job is to cultivate your lane, meaning, the more you discover and develop the space YOU were created to occupy on this planet, the LESS things will remain the same. Accepting is the precursor to correcting.

Accountability: You cannot change that which you do not own. Burying experiences doesn't diminish them, but owning them gives you the power to trade them in for a higher perspective. The more you fight with what happened in your life before, the more of what happened before will grow. Own it. Transmute it. Profit from it.

Allowance: It's ok to feel a range of emotions. It's ok to get frustrated. It's ok to question if you can do this. But DO NOT STAY IN THAT SPACE. A temporary feeling will no longer get in the way of a permanent goal. Allowing yourself to feel how you feel is the best way to honor your present, but processing those emotions and moving ahead is the best way to get to your future.

Action: Just as a body that's developed to run a race, a mind that appraises, accepts and accounts for itself is also ready to allow action to take place. Give thanks for all you've experienced and that you possessed the courage to answer the call to change. Step into your new territory with confidence and as a new you. Command a new life and life will respond in a new way! *

Ready to exercise? Let the stretch begin!

For more content on how you can develop a fit mind, please see the last page of this book for information on my Intrinsic Guidance Offerings.

Accountability Exercises

Exercise One: The Blueprint

So, you want to be made over. You feel out of synch with the life around you and out of touch with the life within you. But WHAT exactly do you want remodeled and WHY? What kinds of thoughts surround your current state of being? Even if you feel unsatisfied with multiple aspects of your life, identifying one specific area to initially reconstruct will help you focus on that space, without wandering off to another before it's completion. You're the architect of your present and future! Instead of relying on a literal blueprint, you're to create a manifesto declaring WHAT you want to make over and WHY redesigning this aspect of you is important! Blueprints aren't general. They are very specific, so be as clear as possible in your manifesto. Make the reason 100% your own; independent of what others say should be fixed about you. Use the lines below to state your manifesto. Duplicate this form so it can be used for each internal space that you're aiming to reshape. Remember: this is your lane and there is NO competition. Diligently address and complete one manifesto at a time. Allow yourself the opportunity for this declaration to become a habit before jumping onto another. Celebrate your diligence daily and watch your desires MANIFEST! New thoughts will become new things!

The words below are my manifesto, my blueprint in words. I will put in the work throughout the day to see that this will come to pass. I am patient, diligent and loving towards myself in this new process.

I will redesign my thoughts around this aspect of my life: -

_____

_____

_____

_____

_____

I am aiming towards a new perspective of this aspect because:

_____

_____

_____

_____

_____

Once my thoughts are redesigned, I have no choice but to experience:

_____

_____

_____

_____

_____

If it was difficult to write the manifesto, fret not. You're venturing into new territory. Be honest and patient with yourself. The architect who draws a blueprint didn't do so overnight nor did the remodeling happen in 24 hours. We're not microwaving this process: slow cooking is the pace for this space.

Exercise Two: The Dig

I can imagine the first picture that popped into your head after reading the name of this exercise. We've all watched home remodeling shows. After they've decided what needs to be redesigned, they call in their crews to DEMOLISH the old space: they tear down walls, break down dilapidated fixtures, and dig up the ground below them to make room for the new design...and you must do the same. Of course, you didn't expect your desires to manifest without allowing a clear mental space for them to be planted, did you?

The Subconscious Mind

Remember those stubborn roots in your parents or grandparents garden that you watched them struggle to pull out the soil? They would work up a serious sweat trying to remove the entire root, so the soil can be treated with new seeds. Heaven forbid they didn't uproot all of them, because if they didn't, the new plants wouldn't stand a chance to bloom. The old roots would occupy the space the new seeds needed to grow, and before they could even get comfortable, the prevailing roots overtook them. The show was closed before it was ever open.

The dig is where we uproot the subconscious mind. It is where our beliefs planted by family, friends, teachers, and media, have lived for so long that without us recognizing, it reigns as pilot of our lives. Many are so oblivious to the power of the deeply rooted, prevailing thoughts they have, they've convinced themselves that the effects of them don't exist. For example, some have a fear of swimming in ocean water, even though they've never stepped foot into an ocean. They want to venture into that territory, but the thought of a piranha or shark attack keeps them at bay. How can one fear something they've never tried? Once they go through the dig, they easily recollect the conversations they heard as a child, about a story a relative told of the person who was eaten by a shark while treading in unknown waters. The story they heard was told with such dramatic images of horror that the person hearing the story subconsciously vowed NEVER to step into an ocean. The vibrational force of that discussion rang deep into the sub consciousness of the child, who is now an adult afraid to go into the ocean.

The subconscious conversations we have with ourselves turn into how we consciously live our lives. The words we hear via a motivational talk, church sermon or audio book lay on the surface, our consciousness, for a little while, which provides that euphoria we feel after leaving service or a power meeting. But unless that belief takes root in our subconscious, IT WILL NOT BLOSSOM. It's the reason so many feel down in the dumps by Monday no matter how powerful Sunday's church message was. The life we want to live will manifest based on what our subconscious says, not based on what our consciousness wants. Our most prevalent thought stems from our subconscious beliefs. The only way to restructure our subconscious is to dig it up. The only way for the old thoughts not to grow back is to offer them a new "food" source (we'll feed them something new in exercise three). In the meantime, let's get prepared for the dig.

There's nothing clean about a dig, but a few things are for certain: you discover things you didn't know existed, you remember things you thought you'd forgotten, and you get cleaned up after it's all done. The dig is directly connected to your manifesto. A new perspective cannot be clearly brought to fruition when the old view is prevalent. An eating habit cannot be reversed or the creation of a new career cannot begin if the reason you don't have those things aren't addressed. Have your shovel and tissue ready but don't forget: what's hidden in the dark always come to light, and the light is here to guide you.

Let's begin in the dark. Find a dim, quiet space in your home for a few moments of daily solitude. If no such place exists within your home, your car or a park will do. The goal is to find a place with as little distraction as possible. LEAVE YOUR CELL PHONES OUT OF THIS SPACE. What we're plugging into has nothing to do with social media, but everything to do with the inner-net.

Address the most prevalent thought in your mind: no need to think too hard about which one. It's that one that keeps you stuck, unhappy, and doubtful about things in your life. It's that old, lingering thought that makes you whisper to yourself, "are things ever going to change?" Yes, that same thought that makes you question if "things" are made to work in your favor is the same thought that relinquishes your control of navigating your reality. That's the thought you are going to work with.

The "5 W's And One H Rule" for a successful dig

In solitude, with your most prevalent thought, ask yourself the series of questions below. The who, what, when, where, why, and how's of the dig help us to finally connect the pieces of our life's puzzle. The purpose of starting in reverse is because we must start on the surface of anything to get to its root. No such tool exists that allows a gardener to uproot the weeds without first inserting it onto the surface, and no such journey towards healing your inside can begin without addressing the thoughts that manifest your current outer reality.

My most prevalent thought/emotion is

_____

_____

_____

_____

_____

HOW has the thought manifested in your daily life and how has it affected your relationships with self/people and/or food?

_____

_____

_____

_____

_____

HOW does this reoccurring thought make you feel?

_____

_____

_____

_____

WHY has it been a challenge to release the thoughts that bring about the unwanted emotions?

_____

_____

_____

_____

_____

WHERE do you always seem to be when you experience the feelings brought upon from this thought?

_____

_____

_____

_____

WHEN is your first memory of this thought?

_____

_____

_____

_____

Once the thought occurs, **WHAT** does it make you feel like doing?

_____

_____

_____

_____

WHAT incident made it become your most prevalent thought?

_____

_____

_____

_____

_____

WHO told you this untruth about you and/or your experience?

_____

_____

_____

_____

_____

WHO do you have to forgive?

_____

_____

_____

_____

_____

Speaking of forgiveness...

F (oster) Forgiveness!

Remember: I am human too. I know it can be a challenge to forgive those who you feel has wronged you. I know you feel if you forgive the person, they are "getting" away with their actions, and I know you think that holding on to a non-forgiving feeling makes them more worthy of punishment. Here's the reality: the experience you had can only be felt by YOU. Holding on to the experience you deem negative will not affect them the same way you're allowing it to affect you. Since we cannot, nor should we desire to change the experience of others, we must use that energy to shift our view of the things that have happened to us.

Forgiveness has nothing to do with getting away with everything. It has everything to do with walking away with the lessons you need to be a knowledgeable man or woman. We cannot change what happened, but we can always change its purpose. Earlier in this book I spoke of things happening FOR us and not TO us; forgiveness is saying "thank you" to the person(s) who delivered the lessons to us. To forgive doesn't mean you like the way the lesson was delivered or the delivery person; it means you understand that the assignment HAD to be given in order for your progression.

So why forgive? Because to *for* (prefix meaning "away") *give* (meaning "granting permission") means you are relinquishing the way you were taught the lesson in order to receive its purpose. You cannot hold on to how you felt while wanting to feel something different at the same time. Both frequencies cannot occupy the same space. Forgiving then becomes the only way to be receptive to what life wants to offer you. Don't take the delivery of the lesson personal, only what's inside of it, and remember even teachers (those who deliver the lesson) get schooled too. Most importantly: forgive yourself. What you knew then has brought you to what you know now. You couldn't have the life you now love without feeling the pain you felt then. It's all on purpose and that purpose is ALL good.

BUT SOMETIMES FORGIVENESS IS NOT ENOUGH

Doing things because someone said so didn't come easy to a "why" child like myself. "Sahsha, eat your peas!" "But why, daddy?" I replied. "Because they are good for you! You're already skinny enough so I need you to eat your vegetables!!" Sounded well meaning, but what was good for me, I thought, were those Twinkies that were waiting for me in the freezer (because who didn't love a near frozen Twinkie) or the pineapple flavored gummy bears that were staring at me from on top the counter asking to be eaten. What's good for me, I felt, was just letting me eat what I wanted to eat because it tastes good! But a parent's job is to attempt to lead children in the "right" direction, whether they follow what's "right" for themselves or not. My job, however, was to ask why until I got my answer, or until my relentlessness prevailed and I was freed from the dinner table because they were tired of fussing with me...or because they didn't know how a pea was really beneficial to me.

In my "adult" mind, peas and forgiveness are alike. It's something we're told to consume or do because it's good for us, but that still doesn't make it easier for us to eat, let alone digest. Even after reading what I wrote above, you still have a hard time believing that forgiving will make you free and without it, you are living a self-imprisoned life. You still see it as the one who committed the "infraction" against you going free without a trial. With that perspective, forgiveness indeed looks like a "get out of jail free" card for the "aggressor", and a harsh sentence for the "wrongly" punished. And you may be thinking that the ones telling us to forgive have forgiveness work to do themselves...so why are you forgiving again?

In order for you to even begin the process of forgiving, you must see how it can benefit YOU first. The importance of forgiving and making it stick must go beyond the promise of it "making you free". Forgiving has to directly translate into a tangible reward for the forgiver, not just something one must ambiguously do. Forgiving must have been experienced with a personal benefit for the forgiver FIRST, before they are willing to give it away to someone who has "wronged" them. Forgiving is not only essential and enlightening, but it's also the best form of escapism from a not so comfortable situation.

Forgiveness is like insurance. We purchase insurance in the event that IF something happens to hurt our property or us, we have coverage to fix or replace it. You never want to use insurance, but it's always good and necessary to have. Why? Because unfavorable situations WILL happen. You will have to invest money (deductible) and processing time (paper work, interviews, etc.) to get through it. But how you're prepared to handle it coupled with KNOWING that whatever was damaged will get fix is what makes insurance worth it. Insurance helps you cover unforeseen circumstances almost guaranteeing you a worthy outcome. Forgiveness can work the same way. Forgiving gives you the ability to process what's happening in a way that ensures you'll get the lesson without the luggage. Forgiveness is full coverage freedom.

But how does one forgive?

Close your eyes.

Imagine the scales of justice. In the middle there's your body, which represents the pedestal. Your arms represent the beam and your hands, the scale. Now, identify your weight, meaning the person and the action they committed "against you" that needs forgiving. Place your weight in your right hand. Let me explain why. In many ancient spiritual practices, even in recent religions like Christianity, the right hand represents *giving away* and in this case, you want to give away whatever burden that's weighing you down. Notice how heavy the weight makes you feel on your right side. You naturally lean more on the side that has more weight, so without knowing it, you're FAVORING the side that creates the most imbalance. You are accommodating the exact thing that is taking up so much unwanted space in your life. Now that's heavy. Look at your right hand. It is filled to the brim and its grip is getting tighter to hold on to your burden. Your body (nature) wants to let go, but your mind's (ego) grip is strong, based on how you've been taught to interpret your encounter. Look at how the weight on your right, your unwillingness to forgive, is manifesting in your life. You are most likely stuck being "right": justifying your feelings as "right", how you think is "right" and how you look is "all right" for someone who's been through what they've been through, based on someone else's action that wasn't "right" ...but how you feel, think and look doesn't display "righteousness". All this wanting to be "right" has you feeling all "wrong". It's time to stop being "right", and start being light! How can you be light?

Go Left.

When we hear the term "going left" we think of someone doing things different from the norm and out of the ordinary. Even when you hear that someone has "left" home, your mind automatically paints a picture of someone going on a unique, personal adventure to develop a part of themselves that couldn't be done "right" where they are. There is power going in the opposite direction of frustration and imbalance. Are you ready to give it a go?

Your left side, according to most Divine practices, is the *receiving side*. This is the side that needs attention and intention. This is the side that has its arms wide open to receive: not the weight from the right, but the lessons brought to light that will open the doors to forgiveness. If the only thing that's keeping the right side alive is the grip we have on it, and if that grip is causing us to tip over on the physical and emotional scale AND if all we must do is allow the experience we're holding on to in the right hand show itself for what it truly is, for it to move to the left, THEN MOVE LEFT. The left can only receive what the right is willing to let go of. The left wasn't made to carry any weight because intrinsically...naturally, its purpose is to receive light. To transmute weight into light, *you must make light of the weight*. Tight grips will always sink ships, so if you intend to truly live, you must give yourself the opportunity to experience the other side of pain. How else can your weight travel to your left side, if not light as a feather? How else can you get to the light if you don't let go of the weight?

Experiences are energy. Once energy is transmuted, it becomes anything you intend it to be. If you are ready to forgive, if for nothing else other than you are tired of the grip that unforgiveness has over your life, loosen up the grip of what's "right". Choose to see how the experience has or can enrich your existence. Has the perceived pain helped you realize what you will not, for example, ignore, tolerate or expect from someone else? Has your weight helped you to see how you have maintained the pain that you've spent years complaining about? Once you begin to pick apart your experience with a new set of eyes, you will begin to see the light in it. As more light is shone, the left side is activated and you begin to receive the original intention of the lesson. Soon the right can become more "upright" as tension is released and the experience is transferred from pain to gain. Before you know it, the right side, what was, and the left side, what is, now reside in harmony. Balance is restored and forgiving can begin.

Repeat the above processes with each dig. As you experience the freedom gained from digging up and resolving thoughts/emotions that used to rule your life, you will confidently and diligently uproot other thoughts that have led to emotions and reactions that no longer serve you.

There is an immense freedom in getting to the root of things. There is an immense freedom in getting to the root of you.

Exercise Three: The Refurbishing

Your slate is just about clean. You've followed your blueprint and completed part of your renovation by tearing down the walls that used to support your old way of thinking, living and eating. The rubble must be removed, however. It's time to clean up the old and redecorate with the new!

The most important part of any structure is its foundation; from the floor, the building is constructed on top of, to the walls that support it, a building, no matter how beautiful it's exterior, will not withstand environmental changes without a solid infrastructure. From the heat of the summer, to the winter's snow, from hurricanes and flash floods to tornado row, the structures that endure it all do so because of what's supporting its interior.

The same rings true for your body temple. It must now be reinforced with words and beliefs that support a renewed you. The dig addressed excavating old thoughts and actions that no longer represent the way you chose to live in the now. The refurbishing is where the subconscious is fed the things you want to see manifest. Feed your mind seeds of prosperity, and your body, soul and life WILL be prosperous!

Earlier in part two, I provided thirty motivations for you to not only get acquainted with talking to yourself in a new way, but to experience the positive outcome the words can potentially have in your life. Now, it's your turn. Are you committed enough to change that you will continue to step out of your comfort zone by writing reinforcements to your manifesto? It's easy to eat clean and speak enlightened when surrounded by those who'll hold accountable, but how accountable are you willing to be with yourself without any outside guidance? This journey ultimately is your own, specifically designed with you in mind. So, it makes sense that most of the words that'll become the soundtrack of your life come from your own unparalleled encounters.

On the lines below, I'd like you to begin rewriting your own script. Create three heart-centered affirmations to repeat multiple times throughout the day, with at least one being about your renewed health goals. The only "rule" to this game is that the motivations must be your own. The length of it doesn't matter, only its depth. The writing is on the wall, but this time it's got YOU written all over it!

Motivation one

_____

_____

_____

_____

_____

Motivation two

_____

_____

_____

_____

_____

Motivation three

_____

_____

_____

By no means should you limit yourself to just three motivations. As you feel the need to "decorate" your subconscious…do so! There can never be enough positive reinforcement within the walls of our minds and once your own custom-made motivations get acclimated to its new conditions, your life has no choice but to shine, and that bright light WILL attract visitors.

Exercise Four: The Grand Opening

It's amazing what can be accomplished when you put your restored mind to it. You have witnessed, by your own doing, a transformation beginning within yourself that you couldn't have previously imagined. How do you feel in your new skin? Still hard to believe this is the start to a new life? Besides "awesome" and even "unsure", can't quite pinpoint how to describe what your feeling? Your life's mission isn't about having all the answers, it's about knowing that because you're asking and acting in your own behalf, the questions you contemplate will lead you further up the path of self-development. The questions you ask to self (The Divine Source) are mere stepping-stones towards the discovery of yet another part of you. You're not the only one who will have questions about this "new" you… so will others.

The Critics

The opinions of others are vast and plentiful. No matter how much thought, effort, and money that was spent on a structural renovation, there will always be a good amount of people who feel the old building was better. They question why the architects and investors felt the need to change if nothing appeared broken. As they walk through the new building, they take issue with not knowing where things are anymore, why the travertine was replaced with marble, and they continually question the motives of those involved in making the changes. Simply put, they just don't like changes!

…And that's ok.

You think, feel and look better than you've ever experienced before. You are now conscious of your thoughts, which make you conscious of your decisions behind every action, including the food you eat. Just like the grand opening of a newly designed building or car, the display of the new you will have people lined up to witness its splendor. Although most will share your excitement and your enthusiasm and even inquire about what you are doing, some just won't like it. There will be some, surprisingly those closest to you that will question the changes. They will find it hard to believe that there was ever a need for you to change because, from the surface, you appeared happy and content. And even after you explain your need to live from a place of authenticity and liberation, they STILL will not be convinced of your intentions. Not because you aren't reflecting a healthier, slimmer, more peaceful you, but because your changes force them to look at the changes they need to make in themselves that they've ignored for FAR too long.

When any aspect of our environment changes, it's a personal call to action. The local grocery store that used to be open 24 hours a day now closes at 9pm. That change makes us have to plan out our shopping schedule in advance as opposed to relying on the convenience of it being open all day and night. The grace period the power company used to offer in paying bills has been revoked, so now you have to manage your money wisely in order to pay your bill on time. As you've done the work to shift your internal and external environment, those closest to you have no choice but to reassess the things they're doing, and not doing for themselves. The responsibility that comes with making changes is a burden most don't want to carry, so as opposed to admiring you or asking you about the steps you've taken in your redesign, they question why you weren't happy with the old one.

See, comfort zones are indeed comfortable, but create complacency. Those cemented to their comfort zones would rather stay in an outdated space than venture into a new one and when they see those around them do a new thing it makes them reflect. Reflection will lead them to that "dark closet" they were taught to run from, so in their comfort zone they will remain. Take nothing no one says or does personal, as it's only a reflection of how they feel about themselves. You have a grand opening to celebrate, and you should do it in style!

You instinctively do some things different now. Whether you used to wake up thinking about the dread of work and bills, and now upon waking you give thanks and declare this day to be the most amazing, writing about the changes makes them that much more real!

On the lines below, list five things that have become automatic as a result of your redesign.

1. _____

_____

_____

2. _____

_____

_____

3. _____

_____

_____

4. _____

_____

_____

5. _____

   _____

   _____

Even though you're on the road towards a deeper renewal, habits, no matter how unbeneficial they are now, take time to break. Not everyone gravitates to the grand opening on day one; neither will new practices become the norm overnight. On the following lines, list the five things you've had to remind yourself to be aware of sine the grand opening.

1. _____

   _____

   _____

2. _____

   _____

   _____

3. _____

   _____

   _____

4. _____

_____

_____

5. _____

_____

_____

No one wants to have to remodel a building or his or her body temple for the same issues that were present before. On the lines listed below, list three things that you will have to do on a more than daily basis in order to maintain your new happy space.

1. _____

_____

_____

2. _____

_____

_____

3. _____

   _____

   _____

Walk that new walk! Talk that new talk! Think that new thought! Celebrate you! There's nothing like embracing your entire journey, tears and triumphs alike!

Part 3

Wellness

I happily and lovingly support myself through the process of self-maintenance.

Chapter 7

On Your Way To Wellness...

The road to wellness will always have its twists and turns, detours and traffic and times when you get to your destination faster than expected. But all of it is contingent upon one thing: having a full tank of gas.

The time that has been taken to get to this point in your journey...the point where your subconscious mind is repositioned to support the life you were born to live, can potentially all be in vein IF you don't continuously support your body temple. How you fill your tank: what you eat, how you cleanse, how you retreat and replenish, and how you choose to move your body, are key components to enjoying life and fulfilling the myriad of goals you have.

The replenishment of your body temple is a collective effort optimized by the utilization of these practices: Freeing your mind with *meditation*. Freeing your body with *detoxification*. Fueling your body with *nutrition*, and flexing your body with *exercise*. Equal maintenance of these supports systems allows each to flourish without neglecting the vital role of another. Exercising your body without the proper foods to propel it, for example is as detrimental as running a luxury car on sub premium gas...it will crash and burn. What you put in your collective body temple will either optimize or obliterate your reality.

Filling your internal well from a holistic standpoint is paramount. No longer will binging on fast foods, excessive shopping and partying or hours in front of the television fulfill you. How you consciously spend your time is in direct correlation to how fast your desires will manifest. Even though you feel and are much more equipped than before to focus on what you want, distractions will still linger, and you must be mindful of them.

Positive Distractions

Have you ever felt a call on your life so strong, that ignoring it was literally like ignoring your own existence? I figured so, especially now that you're in tuned with your inner voice. It still, however, can be an intimidating task to take full control of your life, independent of the influences and realities of others. As a way to delay the necessary self-maintenance needed in a specific area of our growth, we'll often get distracted by excessively engaging in other activities we enjoy for ourselves or others as a way to delay participating in activities that promote our acceleration. *Positive distractions* are positive things you do for yourself or other in excess to avoid addressing the things you KNOW you need to do for yourself. It's a widely accepted belief that people are afraid of failure, but it's also true that some are equally afraid of success, and a great way to avoid it is by doing wonderful, but potentially wasteful things, that aren't a priority to self.

I was a classic enabler. Part my humanitarian nature, and partly because if I didn't help everyone…all the time, I'd be left to do all the little things

I knew I needed to do to catapult my destiny and expedite my success. I made no time to meditate because I used my time taking family and friends everywhere they needed to go without every saying "No" or "I can't right now". I made no time to write because I needed to work out...2 hours instead of 1. I didn't have time to do any entrepreneurial research because I was busy helping my co-workers with theirs...catch my drift? All the things I did were good, but all the time I spent doing them could've been divided into helping them AND supporting myself. Not only did I promote the stagnation of their growth by being their crutch, I delayed my growth under the guise of being a good citizen because I was afraid to see just how GREAT I could become.

I knew what I had to regulate, but how wrong could I be if I allowed imbalance in my atmosphere in order to help others? That thought, I believed, was my saving grace from the inevitable repercussions I'd face by continuously avoiding me. Helping others is awesome, but helping myself was absolutely imperative. Answering emails isn't more important than aligning my emotions. Being a "Yes" man or woman shouldn't supersede saying "No" if needed, and being plugged into social media and all the latest trends takes a back seat to being periodically unplugged from media all together, to make sure I'm all together. Do not be distracted with good deeds. Be attracted to taking the time needed to be great! Fill your cup without fear of overflow, and everyone's thirst will be quenched.

The Well-thy Man

The fruit can only be as strong as the root. Makes sense when we talk about trees and the health of the fruit it bears, but it is also reflected in the very life we live. Take man and woman, (and those who identify as something else) for example. Both are born from the root of a woman, the womb, and their health is determined not only by the condition of the root it spawned from, but the continual maintenance of its temple (both inside and out) after it departs from the womb. However in our current state of affairs men have not been given the "ok" to heal themselves from the emotional baggage that haunts them, but women have. Man is strong, logical, tactical and primary...or so we've been taught. Men are raised to dominate every territory they encounter without emotion or compassion because "it's what men do". Women are left to everything else: nurturing, supporting, maintaining the home and children, mending, working and healing. But what if the one needing all that the woman does is the same dominant man we've all been led to believe needs nothing more than power? How does a man who lives in a world that expects him to support his family support himself? How does a man refill his well?

The woman, the host of all life, is a giver by nature and because of that she is given the opportunity to heal without judgment. As a matter of fact it's expected. Spa parties, retreats, quiet moments and most importantly the chance to cry are societal norms given to us without hesitancy. We are expected to carry our load, heal, and keep moving forward. Men are expected to carry their load and keep moving as well, be the centerpiece of it all, the healing, is not extended to our male complement unless they have reached their breaking point. Only until recently has the emotional and subconscious state of men been a conversation. With the influx of PTSD and an increase in suicide over all racial and economic barriers, attention needs to be given and more importantly permission has to be given to men to heal the parts of them that frequently go ignored. What has to be shifted is when the conversation is had and who has the conversation. In order for us to aid in creating the harmony needed to revitalize the planet and strengthen the union of men and women, women must assist men in healing.

This will be a new territory for most men and there may be some pushback from them when it comes to discussing how they feel. Whether they respond with enthusiasm or not, know that they hear and appreciate what you're saying. Whether it's your mate, friend, co-worker or other family member, letting them know that's it's not only acceptable but mandatory for them to heal themselves from the inside out is vital to the health of them as individuals and us as a collective. We must put a halt to the generational habits of men ignoring how they feel because tradition says they aren't supposed to deal with feelings. Now is the time to encourage men to fill their inner well by seeking counseling, taking up journaling, developing and participating in outreach groups and facilitating conversations about intrinsic wellness. Healing isn't for the weak. Healing is for wellness. We can no longer wait to hear about the next suicide or emotional breakdown of men both older and younger before we act. We must be a shoulder for men to cry on. We must extend our hand, our branches from the tree of life of which the fruit (men) came from, to pull them out of the illusion that men don't have to process pain. And the most fitting person to assist the healing process is their root, the woman.

Meditation By Any Means

Self-awareness is the key that unlocks the door to everything you need, and brings attention to that which you don't. How does one become self-aware? How can you be sure you're following your personal navigation, and not the pre-programmed map we were previously forced fed? The answer is meditation. Meditation is defined as, "to consider as something to be done or effected; Intend; purpose." Meditation then, can be considered the practice needed to effectively manifest your purpose.

How do you begin? Over the years, meditation has gotten the reputation of being a practice solely belonging to Buddhism, Hinduism, or Taoism, but if you believe the definition above to be true, then meditation isn't only for the religious it's for everyone. Is there an ideal time to meditate during the day? I prefer early morning, while the house is still quiet and before newer thoughts bombard my current thoughts, but whatever time you can get it in, is better than not practicing it at all. Meditation is open to serve no matter the time of day, so make no excuses about not having the time. Do not be intimidated by the imagery surrounding meditation. Even though most of us picture someone sitting with their legs crossed and eyes closed as the only way to meditate, there are MANY ways to find your purpose as long as one key component is in place: being present.

Being Present

Remember roll call in class? The teacher would call out each student's name on the roster. Those she called out, who were in class would reply, "here" or "present". Those who were absent obviously, didn't answer. Let's bring this into present day. How can you hear and adhere to your call if you are not aware and present? The only way to hear that which you are asking for in prayer, lamentation or contemplation is in your awareness of the present moment. The primary requirement for meditation is your willingness to practice being still in the present; not thinking about what you want in your future. Being "here" gives you the tools you need to get "there". Being present IS where the idea lives; it's where the magic presents itself. Any other awareness, past or future, is either an elusion of a time that's not meant to be recreated, or an illusion of a time that's yet to be created.

Being present isn't merely a state of physical body; it's a state of mind and a placement of your thoughts. Have you ever been at a social gathering filled with hundreds of people, yet despite the festivities, your mind is elsewhere? In order to fully experience where you are, your body AND mind should be in harmony, otherwise your experience is only a shell of your reality.

The Benefits of Meditation

Can you imagine for a moment the peace that comes with not thinking too much in the past or present, and just absorbing the now? Because meditation provides a pause from your normal more than likely fast train of thought, the benefits of meditation will cause the body and mind a much-needed respite. Dr. Herbert Benson, MD, a Harvard Medical School researcher who in the 1970's conducted research on those who practiced transcendental meditation (that method will be mentioned again later), coined the term "relaxation response" due to the positive, relaxed state of the nervous system of those who were the subject of his study. Since then, research of the "relaxation response" and other benefits, have shown that meditation can temporarily aid in:

- Lower blood pressure

- Improved focus

- Mental clarity

- Less stress

- Slower heartbeat

And from my personal experience, I can link my anxiety with spending too much thought time in the future, while some can connect their depression to dwelling too much in the past. So not only can meditation help regulate the things listed above, it can play a huge part in aiding in anxiety and depression.

So now that you understand the importance of meditation and being present, let's explore some methods of meditation so you can find one that best suits you.

Chapter 8

Meditation Suggestions

Below are a few of many methods you can use to meditate. Whatever your choice, you can start with one method and switch at your leisure. The only commitment you need to make is not in the method, but in the maintenance.

Guided Meditation

Guided meditation is one of the newest meditation methods. It is highly recommended for those who are in the beginning stages of their meditation journey because it offers a "helping hand" during the process. As you sit in a comfortable position, pre-recorded audio containing affirmations to reset your mind, guided imagery to utilize your imagination or instrumental/sounds of nature to promote relaxation serve as the foundation to settle your mind and regulate your breathing. This method is like having a meditation coach to assist you. As your focus begins to strengthen and your desire for deeper meditation arises, you can choose to switch this method for another. A guided meditation I highly recommend is Wayne Dyer's *I Am: Wishes Fulfilled Meditation.*

Mantra Meditation

This type of meditation's primary focus is on…focus. A mantra is a word or syllable, with or without meaning, repetitiously used to create a focused mind. One of the most common mantra's known is "Om". All words have a vibration, and some who practice this form of meditation say a mantra must exude a certain vibrational frequency in order for it to be effective. The one thing that can almost always be agreed on is that repeating the mantra helps the practitioner become unattached from the incessant thoughts that often plague the minds of many. To begin, position yourself in an upright position, spine straight and eyes closed. Silently repeat the mantra during your session. I would suggest committing to at least a five-minute session for starters. The more unattached you get to your thoughts, the more attached you can get to the wonder behind them. With enough practice, the mantra will serve as a "key" to start your meditation, as your unwavering focus will take you through the remainder of your session.

Mindfulness Meditation

The only thing that's on the minds of most is what one should do in the next moment. Realigning our focus towards the present moment is what makes mindfulness meditation, in my opinion, one of the most important meditation practices for our time. As I stated earlier, being present is the only way to know and feel what to truly do next, and the practice of mindfulness helps facilitate that.

Mindfulness meditation is the practice of purposely focusing on the present moment without judgment of whatever feelings, thoughts or emotions that may come up.

Pay attention to your breath. Breathe as deep and as long as you can, homing in on the sensation of breathing itself. Pay attention to your inhale and exhale and how it feels. As you continue, you will become distracted from the sounds outside and the thoughts inside of you and that's ok, just lovingly bring yourself back to your original point of focus, your breath. No matter what, acknowledge how and what you feel in the moment, without judgment. The key to mindfulness meditation is to "be" in, and feel the moment. You can also practice being mindful outside of formal meditation. Taking the time to slowly chew your food, a slow stretch, or a peaceful gaze of the details in your surroundings are others way to make sure you never miss a moment. Being mindful helps you realize that time is always on your side; you've just been too busy to notice it.

There are plenty of other ways to meditate; some are much more intense and traditionally require working with a guru, like Transcendental or Vipassana meditation, while some are so personal it simply requires being alone for 5 minutes, breathing in and out before you run into work or right after you put the kids to bed. Whatever way you choose to meditate, do it and enjoy it consistently. Practice makes perfect and perfecting your way to intention, purpose, and peace is what meditation is all about.

Chapter 9

Detoxification Suggestions

Earlier in this guide we delved into how unhealthy thoughts leads to unhealthy eating habits. Most of us didn't grow up eating clean whole foods as our primary nutrition source, so no matter what or how we're eating now, getting rid of the residual waste of our former ways is of the upmost importance.

When our car gets an oil change, the first thing the technician does is drain out the old oil BEFORE replacing the engine with new oil. Why? Because if the new oil mixes with the old oil, it is now one with the old oil, taking on its properties: filth and non-optimal performance. The new oil will never reach its purpose of lubricating the engine when it's forced to mixed with the old. To reach its desired results, new oil should have a clean slate to penetrate so the engine can receive all of its benefits.

Religious or not, one of the most profound books ever written was *The Bible*. In the gospel, according to Mark 2:22, he states, "And no one pours new wine into old wineskins. Otherwise, the wine will burst the skins, and both the wine and the wineskins will be ruined. No, they pour new wine into new wineskins." Just as new oil or new wine will be like the old if not given clean surroundings, so will your body if not given a proper opportunity to release the old. Detoxification, meaning the "metabolic process by which toxins are changed into more readily excretable substances", can help aid in the release of environmental, food borne or even mental overload, so that your body can easily absorb the nutrients it needs. Detoxing then, isn't a practice that should be done once in a lifetime, but on an as needed basis, when you feel the onset of toxic overload or the desire for a much-needed reset.

Diet vs. Detox

When most people hear the word diet, they automatically think of someone who's eating a certain way to obtain a specific weight goal. When most seek out a diet ONLY for a targeted weight, and not for overall good health, they miss their long-term target. Why? Because it's the intrinsic programming that determines the extrinsic permanency of weight loss. An engine programmed to drive a maximum speed of 80 miles an hour will not go much further than that despite the paint job, tires and body of the car, because its internal make up isn't equipped to support its external appeal. A diet, then, isn't something that should be desired only to secure a specific weight alone; if you want to maintain your best looking and most healthy body temple, you MUST adhere to a diet that's easily processed and its nutrients easily absorbed by your body. Whole, mono or minimal ingredient food with little to no processing involved IS the diet that will not only give you your best health, but your best body. Diet isn't a ten, twenty or thirty-day goal; diet is eating whole foods for a whole life, for the rest of your life.

Detoxing could be considered a support method used in relieving the body from the overload of toxins associated with bad dieting, which can then facilitate the healing process. Whether the toxic source comes from food, environment, drugs, (both legal and illegal) or emotions, detoxing provides an opportunity for your body to recoup from the intake of excessive waste. Detoxing is beneficial not only to those who don't have the best eating habits, but it's also good for those who eat "clean" because we are all susceptible to the side effects of air pollution, processed foods (even if they're not consumed at a high rate) and emotional stress.

Since I've began eating a whole foods, plant based diet, I don't feel the need to detox more than once or twice a year simply because I feel good more often than not. But I'm aware that all things need maintenance, including me, in order to be at my best. The key thing to remember is that diet is daily and detoxing is periodical. The cleaner you eat, the less you have to maintain. "Let thy food be thy medicine" should be the norm, not boundless detoxing or random dieting due to innutritious foods you eat. Eating clean or detoxing for vanity's sake alone will never give you the piece of mind you are seeking because what you're truly seeking goes beyond how you look and dives into the depths of how you feel. How you look and how long you maintain it is the by-product of the continuum of a whole foods diet and a regular state of happiness. Although I'm a huge advocate of detoxing, it should never be looked at as a substitute for a healthy diet.

Fasting

Fasting isn't just for those who "give up" something in order to receive something they want, or for those who adhere to a specific religious doctrine, fasting is defined as the abstinence of all foods, period (not water; always drink water). Many people take to fasting as a way to give their bodies a much-needed break so it can process the foods eaten throughout the days without interference. Fasting is now being received by some in the medical field as a great way for your body to rest, so it can recover. People have put their own twists on fasting; to mean just a general break from something they tend to overindulge in. The popular term, "Meatless Mondays" is a way to fast from eating meat for a day so that our bodies can digest the meat previously consumed (often in excess). You can fast from sugar, alcohol, or fast foods for a day, week, or month, whichever you see fit. *Intermittent fasting* is fasting that is done for a period of time within the same 24-hour period. Most of us fast daily and don't realize it. The time between our last meal of the evening and our first meal of the next day to BREAK the FAST (breakfast) is a period of fasting! It takes about 6 to 8 hours to digest a meal from stomach to intestines, so you can see how three meals a day can put high demands on our bodies, in addition to everything else it does for us. Fasting helps our bodies do their jobs so we can do ours.

The Victorious Detoxer

Slow and steady wins the lifelong race, especially when starting something new. Those who've successfully completed any detox have implemented:

1. Mental Fortitude – Challenges are begun, maintained and won in the mind. Prepare yourself for the task ahead by remembering your purpose and envisioning positive results.

2. Hydration – Often times when we think hunger is calling, it's thirst. In order to keep your head in the game and to aid in the release in toxins, drink plenty of water, a gallon a day if possible, or at least half your body weight in ounces. You weigh 160 lbs.? Drink at least 80 ounces of water daily.

3. Meal Prep – No one goes on vacation without preparation; where to sleep, what activities to participate in, and air accommodations are all made in advance, and so should you prepare your meals before you begin detoxing. Shop for your groceries the day before the detox and replenish your fruit and vegetable supply before they run out to ensure that you don't "slip" up and eat foods that don't support your detox.

4. Self-Care – To be successful during any change one must take care of the temple that is hosting the change. While you're detoxing indulge in a facial, massage, infrared sauna session or a colonic to aid in the passage of toxins and to help you enjoy your wellness adventure.

What To Expect While Detoxing

Since we're speaking of detoxing, I'm not going to sugarcoat anything (pun intended). The premise of this guide is to prepare you to shift from a state of chaos to a state of calm. Nature shows us that after every storm, no matter its length, there is a calm...but we must whether the storm!

Regardless of the method you choose, detoxing calls for a temporary pause on the foods you regularly consume, and that can be a shock to your routine. Just as some babies resist solid food when being weaned, the first couple of days detoxing will bring about different levels of resistance within you. Your body is releasing toxins so if you're feeling a little uncomfortable in the beginning, it's a good sign that the detox is doing what it's meant to do! You can never anticipate your exact reaction, but some people initially experience: Headaches, mental and physical fatigue and irritability. On the flipside, as the detox progresses and subsequently ends, many experience increased energy, mental clarity, physical and emotional weight release, regulated bowel movements, clearer skin and an overall feeling of vitality, focus and improved health.

The Many Ways To Detox: Which one is for me?

The amount of advice out there can be a bit overwhelming when you dive into the pool of information on anything health related. The best way to know which method suits you is to follow the ones that resonate with your inner core the most. I have tried a few detoxification methods and I have two listed below that you can start with and progress into. From a one-day detox to a twenty-day detox and beyond, start where you know you can finish initially, as completing one task gives you the confidence to finish another. Please consult with your physician before starting any detox or fast.

Juice/Smoothie Detox

This particular detox involves drinking freshly squeezed, extracted or blended fruits and vegetables (herbs may be added for taste variations and extra health benefits) throughout the pre-determined amount of detox days. This detox rarely includes pre-packaged, store bought juices and smoothies you find in the grocer's isle, but may include fresh, local, cold pressed juices and smoothies found in your store's refrigerator section. Buying juices can get expensive, so it's always best to purchase a juicer, blender or extractor of your own not only for financial reasons, but to get the most nutrition from this detox. The fresher the juice, the more active the enzymes and minerals are in the juice that your body can effectively absorb for ideal healing. Many gravitate towards this detox because it's a sure-fire way to get all the nutrients their body needs in a delicious way without having to "taste" the vegetables. It may sound petty, but the reality is some people haven't developed a taste for vegetables because they just haven't eaten enough of them. Although eating vegetables are best, it's still highly beneficial to consume your veggies via juicing, then to not consume them at all.

Herbal Supplement Detox

To eat nutritious is one (great) thing, but to take in nutrition while getting help releasing wasteful build up is another! We can never truly understand the amount of toxicity we've absorbed over our current lifespan until we release it. Feeling is believing and being sluggish is NOT normal! Detoxing while taking herbal supplements to reset your major body systems such as your lymphatic (lymph nodes, spleen, tonsils, etc.) cardiovascular (heart, blood, blood vessels) respiratory (lungs, trachea diaphragm, etc.) and digestive systems (liver, pancreas, gallbladder, stomach, small and large intestines, etc.) will not only assist in resetting the individual systems, but will facilitate a highly functioning body unit! Our body isn't a home of separate systems whose mission is independent of the other; our body is one unit whose purpose is to maximize our lives, one healthy system at a time. When one system isn't at its best, the other ones, to a degree, can suffer, and this type of detox can help in making sure that all systems are working at its best.

Many gravitate towards these types of detoxes because it doesn't exclude eating! Chewing is a not so recognized comfort that most enjoy, (because eating is a huge part of our lives) and it's where digestion begins. If you can't go without chewing and it's important to reset your vital body systems, this type of detox is made for you. Each detox has its dietary rules to follow, so I suggest starting one whose rules you're ready to adhere too. I highly recommend The 20 Day Full Body Detox (see reference page for details), but there are many out there for you to choose from.

After the detox...

You've experienced amazing results. After weeks of cleansing your body and strengthening your mind, the last thing you want to do is go back to your old ways of eating and feeling. Grocery shop the same way you did while you were detoxing, gradually introducing yourself to certain foods to see if they are a "fit". Listen to your body, as it will tell you what it wants and what it doesn't. *Do not force old wine (eating habits) into new wineskin (a renewed body).* Detoxing cleans your pallet so to speak, so many experience an internal shock of sorts when they attempt to eat like they did before. Consuming large amounts of simple carbohydrates found in candy, soda and a number of processed foods, sends your bodily systems into sprint mode, when it had been used to running a steady race. Remember: you did not detox for temporary results. You cleansed in order to aid your body in resetting itself to its natural state of being so it can thrive off nature, meaning less processed, more progress.

Detoxing of the mind, spirit, and body temple are important steps in maintaining the life shift you've worked so hard to begin. Once you detox, you begin to feel the definition of alive! Aches, pains, and fatigue can be a thing of the past if you no longer consume the things that brought them on! Releasing toxins from your body will make nutrition more useful and exercise perhaps more endurable.

Chapter 10

Nutrition Suggestions

Our minds are open; our bodies are ready, but are YOU ready to bid farewell to your old way of eating that isn't meant to serve the renewed you? Unlike meditation, detoxing and exercise, eating is the one thing you're trained to do on a daily basis, so what you eat is pivotal to your everyday holistic successes.

What time's the right time to eat?

Perpetual education has taught you that you should eat three meals a day, with your biggest meal being at dinnertime. When we think of meal portions, the familiar vision of a breakfast filled with eggs, bacon, pancakes, sausage, cereal, milk and orange juice typically starts the day and dinner consisting of steak, potatoes, chicken and pasta in cream sauce usually ends it. Lunch is typically similar to dinner, but a slightly smaller portion.

According to livestrong.com, a 2013 study published in *Obesity Research* shows that those who consumed their biggest meals before 3 pm released more weight than those who ate their biggest meal after 3 pm, with both groups consuming the same amount of calories per day.

Another study measured how insulin, a hormone that plays a major role in converting the sugar in our food into energy, was harder to process during evening hours as opposed to active hours, meaning that food sugars which provide our bodies energy is best processed when we are the most active: during the day.

I eat my biggest meal during midday, when the sun is at its highest and when I utilize the most of my energy. If my food is best metabolized when I'm most active AND if I don't eat a big meal in the evening (when the sun and my body are preparing for rest), I sleep well and wake up energized. As a matter of fact, I tend to have some pretty crazy dreams if I eat too heavy, too late. My goal is to put as less stress on my body and its systems as possible, feel my best, and not pick up any added weight during the process, so what works for me is eating my biggest meal at high noon, or before 5 pm. I follow the sun! I eat when it's at its peak so I may be at mine. When it's about to rest, I don't eat. Don't take my word for it. Eat your biggest meals at various times of the day and see when you feel and look your best. Practice this to get the results that suit you best, without knocking yourself if you "slip". If you make healthy habits the norm, that normal will support you when abnormal occurs. This journey isn't about knocking yourself when you have a misstep; it's about bouncing back on your path and turning the misstep into a two-step…forward.

The "Five W's and one H Rule" to maintaining nutrition

During the accountability exercises, we went over (in reverse) the who, what, when, where, why and how's of our most prominent thoughts in order to get to their root cause. The same structure can be used in not only examining your eating habits, but in maintaining them.

Let's now use these questions to focus specifically on diet and nutrition.

WHO told you what foods should and shouldn't be enjoyed?

Answering this will help you identify the source of your diet challenges and it'll allow you to examine how those views affected the ones who held them as well.

WHAT is or was the main reason you had apprehensions towards changing your diet for the better?

WHAT do you look forward to from eating in a new way?

Answering these questions will help you identify if your reasoning came from, for example, the fear of something new or social conditioning, etc. and it will help you keep your focus on your present goals.

WHEN where you first told what's an acceptable diet to maintain?

WHEN did you begin getting questioned about the changes in your diet?

Answering these questions will help you remember how long you've been subjected to the beliefs of others and why you haven't been able to commit to sound dietary changes.

WHERE would it be the most challenging for you to adhere to your new diet?

Answering this can help prepare you before you go out with family or friends, or before going to work, especially if the people closest to you eat in another way.

WHY do you feel you cannot commit to a diet that will fuel the life you are now preparing to live?

Answering this can determine if your hesitation towards making healthy dietary changes possibly stems from your subconscious fear of future successes and it can also highlight the trend you potentially have of not completing projects or committing to long term goals.

HOW will eating a new way facilitate the successful completion of your health and overall life goals?

Answering this will allow you to follow the blueprint you made during the Accountability Exercises. It will also reconfirm within you that eating well means living well.

The "Eating Clean" Stigma

When people hear the term "eating clean" they cringe, and I get it: that term, like many that become a trend, can lose its power due to oversaturation. What is clean eating? Is it a matter of opinion? Eating clean is supposed to mean eating in way that involves minimally processed food with no artificial ingredients. Eating clean isn't exclusive to a certain type of diet. Eating clean can be applicable to meat eaters, pescatarians, vegetarians, vegans, those who follow a paleo diet, and fruitarians alike. The term eating clean, as we know it, is independent of WHAT you eat, per se; it's in HOW it's prepared, WHAT it consists of, and WHERE it comes from. Makes sense, right? I'd like to challenge you to make this term, if it's one you choose to use, even easier.

When you hear the word "clean," you presumably think easy to navigate, welcoming, uncomplicated, inviting and most importantly, simple. If that rings true to you, is how you're eating truly clean? Was there a process involved with your food that included more than a few minutes of prep or no prep time at all? Does the food easily travel through your system without rendering you sluggish or lethargic? Can you simply pick, rinse and eat your food? Does your food need massive amounts of heat to be palatable? These questions aren't to persecute you, but to jog your consciousness about the words you use and if they're at all applicable to your life, or just a figment of the life you want to live. If you desire to eat clean remember this sentiment: Eating clean is eating in a way that is simple to prepare, simple to attain, easily digestible, easily excreted, easily pronounced, easily chewable, non-life-threatening, promotes longevity, demotes planetary wear, promotes energetic responses, and tastes good without any additives. Eating clean isn't complicated. If you can't easily pronounce what you're eating, your body can't easily process it. Additives add weight to you. Preservatives preserve your current state, or prevent you from expanding to a higher one. LISTEN TO THE WORDS! The awesome thing is that you can begin to eat in a "clean" way RIGHT NOW no matter what your last bite of food consisted of! Learn to tune into your body as you eat because it will tell you what's best for it.

I'll never forget when I stopped eating meat the second time around. I love homemade tacos and as a "healthy" substitute, I ate a lot of ground turkey with my tacos, Italian dishes, and chili. Whether I wasn't tuned into my body before or it was simply fed up, I started to have extreme indigestion shortly after its consumption. I initially thought it was the gluten in the spaghetti and tortillas that caused my discomfort, so I eased up from eating those for a while, but to no avail; as soon as I consumed ground turkey again, my unwelcomed companion indigestion was right there. I accepted soon after having indigestion for the umpteenth time that I had to part ways with ground turkey, but that didn't mean parting ways with my favorite dishes. I discovered a soy substitute, then a pea protein substitute, to now eating tacos with walnut meat (yes, you heard correctly, walnut meat). Not only do I not feel deprived, I no longer have indigestion all because I paid attention to my body and happily sought an alternative.

I'm a non-meat eater, but it took me some time to get there. First, I eliminated chicken and red meat, then seafood (I was never a big seafood eater), then cheese and finally eggs. Although I'm a plant-based advocate, my job isn't to force you to stop eating animals and animal by-products; my job is to inform you to listen and love your body, eat and shop well informed, do what's best for your body and environment (not your comfort), and to keep life, including diet, simple. I pray the lane you're in leads you to consume a plant-based diet someday, but in the meantime honor where you are and do not intentionally detour from your path because you're afraid to change your eating habits. Welcome the opportunity for change to take place. The journey that's meant for you will NEVER leave you void of enjoyment, even if it looks and tastes different than what you're used to.

Meal Prep

In chapter 10 I spoke of meal prepping in order to be successful during a detox. Meal prepping: preparing your meals in advance in order to maintain your new way of eating, can be a beneficial practice during ANY stage of your journey. Meal prepping helps ensure that you build the confidence needed to adhere to a healthy diet and it can help you survive workplace or happy hour temptations.

For those who have a 40-hour plus workweek, I suggest preparing your meals the day before you go back to work, for the entire week. Slice up those veggies, peel those fruits, make and marinate that salad dressing and steam that quinoa! All you have to do after that is pack and eat! Perhaps you have a catered event to attend and you're not sure what the menu will have for you? Eat a fulfilling meal prior to stepping out so you can feel nutritionally satisfied without feeling "left out" from a social aspect. You can always check the menu of the place you're dining at before you go, so you know your options beforehand.

I Get SO Emotional...So I Eat!

When your cup is empty, you fill it with water. When you're thirsty, you drink it. When your internal well is empty you fill it with...food? In the modern world, food is directly linked to emotions, even more than hunger. Those that find it a challenge to eat clean are more than likely those who have a hard time release "dirty" old thoughts. Certain foods, like sugar and salt temporarily satiates your unaddressed emotion imbalances. Sugar releases *beta-endorphins*. Beta-endorphins are an endorphin produced by the pituitary gland that is a potent pain suppressant. I consumed enormous amounts of sugar because I was attempting to suppress pain, and since sugar was often given to me as a child as a reward or for celebratory reasons, eating sugar for me gave me reasons, albeit them short lived, to be happy. Do you indulge more in salty, crunchy foods? Eating high amounts of salty crunchy foods can be linked to feeling angry, stressed, or resentful. That "salty" feeling has its root and eating salt will only satisfy it for a moment.

Emotional eating soothes a temporary fix; just a drinking creates a temporary buzz, and running, either for exercise or from issues, creates a temporary deterrent. When you clean up you your thoughts, your desire for food will come from a clear place of thinking and feeling. Simplified nutrition will lead to a simplified life. It doesn't get much "cleaner" than that.

Thinking about going meat free?

You're not alone! According to some statistics, it shows that over 7 million Americans are vegetarian, 1 million are vegan, and over 22 million are vegetarian inclined. As being meatless is slowly becoming the new "normal" more people are exploring the options and benefits of minimizing or eradicating all together meat and its by-products. As the minds of many are starting to travel outside of traditions and into the realm of understanding that they have full control of their health, more information is becoming evident that you DO NOT need meat or ANY of its outgrowth to sustain health, feel amazing, and look like your best self.

"Your best self" isn't the same for everyone. For ladies, some are more naturally curvy and some, more lean. For men, some have more natural muscle mass and some do not. No matter your natural disposition, going meat free will help accentuate your natural assets while shedding excess fat. It is true that no matter how hard you try, you cannot control what parts of your body release fat, but considering that excess fat, especially around the stomach area can lead to heart disease, it's safe to say that no matter where the fat exits from, it's alright.

But I Like What I Like!

You love pizza, tacos, burgers and your creamy sauces...yeah, I know. Who doesn't? But just because you like a thing doesn't mean you should have it all the time and certain foods are no exception. But if the need for speed, meaning fast food type delights are calling your name, perhaps you can opt for a healthier, plant based option. Below are two of my favorite go to, plant based indulgences that are equally as tasty and a lot healthier than their popular counterparts. And they are completely raw and detox friendly. Walnut meat has the taste and texture of ground meat and is great for plant based tacos, nachos and enchiladas. The raw vegan "cheese" sauce packs a major punch and can be used on almost anything, and because its nutrient dense, even on salad!

Walnut Meat (serves 2)

2 c. organic walnuts, raw

½ tsp. sea salt

1 tsp. walnut, avocado or grape seed oil

½ tsp. onion powder

½ tsp. cumin

A pinch of cayenne pepper

A pinch of garlic powder

Add all ingredients to food processor. Blend until texture becomes like ground meat. Add to corn tortillas, salad, or lettuce cups and enjoy!

Raw Vegan "Cheese" Sauce

1 c. organic raw cashews

1.5 c. spring water

2 tsp. nutritional yeast

1 c. pimientos

1 tsp. lemon juice

½ tsp. sea salt

¼ tsp. onion powder

Place raw cashews in 3 cups of water to soak for at least 4 hours. The longer they soak, the creamier the texture of the sauce. Drain water. Add cashews, fresh spring water and all other ingredients to food processor and blend until desired texture. If it's too thick, add water. If it's too thin, add a few more cashews. Serve and enjoy!

Well…What About Protein?

Amino acids are the building blocks for protein, and protein is found in MANY plant and plant-based foods. Contrary to popular beliefs, you do not need to eat protein belonging to another animal in order to have strong muscles! If plant food digests easier through our system than flesh does, wouldn't it be safe to at least ponder that plant protein would digest easier, and be absorbed easier in our systems as well?

Wild animals that are carnivores thrive off the consumption of flesh by eating their prey as is, meaning they do not kill the flesh and then drag it over the fire in order to eat it. They consume the flesh as raw as possible to attain the same nutrients the animal thrived off when it was alive. Humans thrive off eating foods that can be consumed "as is", as well, meaning we retain more nutrients when we eat food in its original form. I'm not saying we must only eat our foods raw, I'm saying it would behoove us to consume foods in a state that's most like its original from (minimally cooked) so our bodies can absorb its maximum amount of nutrients. Clothes don't serve the same purpose if they are burned before wearing them. Hair that's overly processed has limited styling and growth potential, and overly processed foods just don't seem like they will provide the quality of protein your looking for, because ALL processes changes things. If you have to heat up your protein source in order to consume it, how much protein is your body really absorbing? I'm no scientist, but if heat changes the structure of almost anything, why isn't easy to believe that it can change the performance of nutrients, particularly protein?

Where To Get Your Protein

Unlike the previously discussed carnivores, gorillas, cows, elephants and giraffes are just a few herbivores that were made to consume and thrive off plant life. Many would argue that humans are made to eat meat while some would debate we've adapted to the ability to digest it. Either way, the one thing you can't debate is the abundance of protein in plant foods!

Below is a chart that highlights not only the amount of protein per serving in beans, grains, and vegetables; it also shows the amount of cholesterol (high cholesterol levels because heart dis-ease, strokes, etc.) per serving and the serving size needed to obtain said amount of protein. Health is WHOLE-stic: if your desire is to serve your body, you must be mindful of all the nutrients your body needs, as a body doesn't thrive on protein alone. Eat in a way to serve your entire body, and your entire body will serve you.

Sources of Plant Protein

Source	Amount of Protein per serving (grams)	Amount of Cholesterol per serving	Serving Size
Grains			
Quinoa	8g	0	185g (1 cup)
Spelt	11g	0	194g (1 cup)
Kamut	11g	0	172g (1 cup)
Brown Rice	5g	0	195g (1 cup)
Wild Rice	7g	0	164g (1 cup)
Beans			
Garbanzo Beans	12g	0	240g (1 cup)
Lentils	18g	0	198g (1 cup)

Sources of Plant Protein

Source	Amount of Protein per serving (grams)	Amount of Cholesterol per serving	Serving Size
Beans			
Pinto Beans	15g	0	171g (1 cup)
Black Beans	14g	0	240g (1 cup)
Seeds/Nuts			
Pumpkin Seeds	12g	0	64g (1 cup)
Walnut	24g	0	100g
Brazil Nuts	14g	0	100g
Hemp Seeds	11g	0	30g
Almonds	22g	0	100g

Sources of Plant Protein

Source	Amount of Protein per serving (grams)	Amount of Cholesterol per serving	Serving Size
Vegetables			
Spinach	3g	0	100g
Broccoli	4g	0	148g (1 cup)
Swiss Chard	2g	0	100g
Dandelio n Greens	3g	0	100g
Kale	3g	0	100g

This chart is only to be used as a tool that will continue to open your mind space. Please consult with your physician before making any dietary changes. Study outside the box. Listen to your body. Eat simply. Enjoy your food and NEVER ignore the urge to do something different if it can lead to a different, healthier, more vibrant you.

Chapter 11

Exercise Suggestions

Move It Or Lose It! The Importance Of Exercise

The body is our mode of transportation. It's a divine vessel gifted to us in order to fulfill our life's mission. Legs are made to walk and run. Arms are made to lift and bend. Toes are meant to flex and stabilize. Abdominal and core muscles are meant to be contracted and strengthened and NONE of this can be done without movement. Our bodies, amongst other things, are made for usage according to their nature. If you purchase or pick vegetables and don't eat them, they go to waste. If you purchase a car and never drive it, it will rust. The same goes for the muscles in our bodies. If you don't use them, they will wither away, rendering you immobile. Atrophy is defined as "a wasting away of the body or of an organ or part as from defective nutrition or nerve damage." And "degeneration from disuse."

The definition above clearly states the importance of not only fueling your body with proper nutrition, but how it can't serve you efficiently if you don't use it. Our bodies are machines that are made for movement just houses are made for shelter. In fact our bodies are a combination of the two; a storehouse for our spirit/energy, thoughts and organs as well as the vehicle needed to expand and nurture the aforementioned.

Thinking positive thoughts and feeding your body whole food nutrition without habitually moving your body temple is simply not inclusive, and remember, you are no longer participating in habits of self-neglect. You must move your body.

The saying "Age ain't nothing but a number" couldn't be more true when it comes to exercise. Some of the sharpest and fittest people I know belong to the generation known as "baby boomers". Some of the unhealthiest people I know are under the age of 30. The correlation I make is whoever moves their body the most frequently feels the best. Many younger people are stuck: behind their desks, in front of their computers or in front of their televisions. Many elders have more control AND appreciation of their time, and use it to add quality years to their life. Simply put; movement keeps your life moving. Immobility keeps you stuck. Make a choice. Make no excuses.

No Time To Exercise, You Say?

You live a busy life and so do I. We both manage to get almost all we need to get done by allotting time for the things we feel are important. Being that we are all given the same 24 hours in a day, let's look at how you can make time to exercise.

Waking up early – Sleep is an important element of our day. Getting insufficient amounts of sleep can determine how the remainder of our day plays out. Getting up 30 minutes earlier to get a quick workout in before you start your day can give your day and your attitude an added boost! Exercise releases endorphins, which positively affect your outlook. Furthermore, exercise promotes deep breathing. Nothing like deep breathing to clear out stale air and stale emotions linked to your potential workday ahead. A little exercise before the kids wake up and soon you won't desire coffee to get your day started!

During Lunch/Break/Children's Naptime – This is where meal prepping is really beneficial! The hour you use to go to your car, drive for food, drive back to work, get back to your desk and THEN eat could be used for eating your prepped meal and taking a leisurely...or brisk walk. If you use the entire hour to eat lunch, use those two 15 minute breaks you get to walk. Whatever you do, get from behind that computer and move around. To my hard working, multi-tasking stay at home moms and dads: you have time and its called naptime! When the little ones are resting is the perfect time for you to be moving. Do a couple rounds of jumping jacks, pushups, and squats or pop in your favorite workout DVD and work your body while you have the time.

The Right Time Is The Nighttime

I can hear it now, "By the time the evening comes around, I'm so tired!" What better way to ensure a great nights' sleep than to put in a little exercise time before you hit the sack? No, you don't have to go to the gym, but you CAN commit to the same type of workout you would during lunch or your children's naptime. Whether with a friend or furry companion, an evening stroll will serve you both well.

The Challenge with Challenges

It's the beginning of a new year. It's the first day of summer. It's Fall solstice. It's a milestone birthday. Whatever the special occasion may be the masses are always motivated when they know it's time to make a significant change. The latest trend to drive people to adjust their diets and lifestyles are challenges.

Whether it's a 10-day challenge where you eat all raw foods, a 20-day challenge where you omit all sugar and caffeine, or a 30-day challenge where you participate in specific workouts, challenges have been touted as a great way to get people moving along a healthier path. But what happens when the challenge is over?

The challenge with challenges is that it offers various support mechanisms prior to and when the event has started. Facebook groups, daily emails and weekly meet ups are the norm during the process. Participants get used to someone holding him or her accountable for eating and exercising according to protocol. Once the challenge has ended and the daily check-ins cease, many participants fall off the wagon because they no longer feel part of the unit that started the mission and they don't believe they are strong enough to continue the mission alone. It is highly important for one to begin a challenge based on their own desire to change, but it is equally important for the organizers; people who assumedly been through the physical and emotional rollercoaster that can come with challenges, to provide post challenge support.

Support is one of the key components in maintaining a new lifestyle, especially when the mind is still getting used to the concept of change. We are heavily enthusiastic at the beginning of anything new, but as time passes and the reality kicks in you may become tempted, unmotivated and unfocused. Your enthusiasm fades and you become unsure and uncomfortable with the road ahead.

Just as a physical therapist sticks around until you have regained bodily strength and just as most rehabilitation centers are there to support their clients after treatment because they understand that people need continual support until their new habits become deeply rooted within them, challenges would benefit participants more effectively if they offered "after challenge support." Whether it be paid consultations, publications, e-courses or workshops, if you join a challenge make sure to participate in one that offers support after the "race" is done. If you feel the need for additional support, do not hesitate to hire a nutrition, life or health coach to give you the continual support you need. If none of those are an option, form a post-challenge support group with your team members where you call or email each other at least once a week to make sure everyone is on track. There are many ways to ensure success and having support is one of them. Before you begin any challenge, make sure your aim is set and your focus is clear so you can hit your long and short-term target.

The Way You Move

Most are pretty particular about the type of coffee they order; they've tried multiple combinations before they found the flavor(s) that tastes best to them. It goes for exercises, as well. Those who say they don't like exercising are really saying they don't like the exercises they've tried. You owe it to yourself to try a variety of moves before you conclude that you don't like to move, just as you'd try on multiple pairs of shoes until you found the right ones. According to the Mayo Clinic, it's recommended to get 150 minutes of moderate exercise a week, broken down, that's 25 minutes a day, 6 days a week. The recommendation doesn't say you have to do the same type of exercise, so get creative with your exercise time and choices! Below is a chart that shows a variety of exercises and how many calories you may burn while participating in them, based on body weight.

Exercise Chart

30 minutes of activities	160 pounds	200 pounds
Activities	Weight of Person and Calories Burned	
Aerobic Step Training	256	317
Aerobics (Water)	146	182
Basketball	292	368
Bicycling	146	182
Bowling	109	147
Dancing	160	200
Gardening	144	180
Golfing	160	200
Hiking	217	273
Jogging (5 mph)	296	370
Jump Roping	456	570

Exercise Chart

30 minutes of activities	160 pounds	200 pounds
Activities	Weight of Person and Calories Burned	
Stair Master	256	320
Swimming	192	240
Tai Chi	146	182
Tennis	282	364
Walking (3.5 mph)	160	200
Weightlifting (free Weights)	109	138
Zumba	190	240

Exercise doesn't only mean "mental or bodily exertion..." it also means "putting into action." Exercise your right to move your body in a direction that will bring you great health, mental clarity, and the discovery of pleasures in unexpected places. All you have to do is commit to MOVEMENT. Your life will thank you for it.

Things to Remember

You've made it to the end of this book, but far from the end of your journey. As you continue up the road to wellness, here are some important things to remember:

- **Know your worth:** you were born for greatness and greatness begins when you're ready to leave mediocrity behind. You deserve better than your previous experiences. Optimal fitness is yours, intrinsically.

- **Seek change from the inside out:** vehicles, technology…and you are maintained from the loving care and attention given to its unseen parts. Nurture yourself holistically: spirit, mind, and body temple.

- **Excavation is a necessary part of life:** getting to the root of each of our emotional triggers is where freedom lies. Embrace the pain in your "dark closet" in order to live in the light. Dig up your old thought processes and replace them with new, life giving emotions, ideas and perspectives. Life isn't a set of punishments; it's a set of possibilities.

- **Keep life simple:** complication is not normal. Once this truth is accepted, life becomes simple and thoughts become less complicated. Forgive. Be responsible. Eat simply. Enjoy good health. It's just that simple.

- **Practice patience:** starting the journey isn't like starting a race. Your lane was made specifically for you, so there's no competition. Make choices that will take you further along your desired path. Expand and maintain your space and enjoy the ride.

- **Move your body:** You have your lane; you have your vehicle, now keep it feeling and looking its best. Experiment with exercises until you find the one that resonates with you. Whatever you do, don't stop moving.

Sweeter than any dessert I've ever eaten, life is the sweetest, most deliciously rich treat I've tasted. In the closet lies my discovery. In the sun lies my energy. On my plate lies my therapy. On this journey lies my directory. In these words, lies our unity.

I've read *The Well*...so now what?

Glad you asked. Embarking on a new personal journey can be frightening, no matter how necessary it is. My job as an Intrinsic Wellness Guide is to aid you in exploring the parts of yourself that you tend to ignore, yet need the greatest amount of attention. This book is a great place to start and return to, but I have more to offer those who are ready to jump deeper into their well.

My Intrinsic Wellness Guidance packages are geared towards multiple levels of readiness.

The Well-Come Hour – is best suited for someone who needs guidance removing their fear of change while getting a general idea of what mindset is holding them back.

The Live Well Package – is intended for those who are ready and committed to having me guide them in uprooting all of their subconscious blocks while creating a blueprint for success in every area in their life.

The Well-th Guidance Circle – are for those who desire to take the journey to intrinsic wellness with a group of enthusiastic, like-minded, accountability-oriented individuals.

I would love to partner with you on this life-changing journey. For more information on how we can work together and for more on my guidance packages, publications and speaking engagements, please visit www.lifeandlightlessons.com andwww.sahshacampbell-garbutt.com.

Follow me on social media:

Facebook @sahshacampbellgarbutt

Instagram @lifeandlightwellness

Twitter @lifeandlight1

In Life And In Light...

#radiatelovenow

References

Dienstmann, G. Types of Meditation – An Overview of 23 Meditation Techniques. Retrieved from http://liveanddare.com/types-of-meditation/#disqus_thread

Beckerman, J. (reviewed by, 2015) Tips To Keep Your Cholesterol In Check. Retrieved from http://www.webmd.com/cholesterol-management/guide/cholesterol-basics

M.D, Picco, M. (2012) Digestion: How Long Does It Take? Retrieved from http://www.mayoclinic.org/digestive-system/expert-answers/faq-20058340

M.D, Laskowski, E. How Much Should The Average Adult Exercise every day? Retrieved from http://www.mayoclinic.org/healthy-lifestyle/fitness/expert-answers/exercise/faq-20057916

Adapted from: Ainsworth BE, (2011) -Mayo Clinic Staff. Activities/Calories Burned. Retrieved from http://www.mayoclinic.org/healthy-lifestyle/weight-loss/in-depth/exercise/art-20050999?pg=2

(2012) Top 25 inspirational quotes by Olympic athletes. Retrieved from http://blog.shareitfitness.com/2012/inspirational-quotes/

Vegetarian Times Staff. Vegetarianism In America. Retrieved from http://www.vegetariantimes.com/article/vegetarianism-in-america/

Bruso, J. (2015). What Should Be Your Biggest Meal? Retrieved from http://www.livestrong.com/article/469196-what-should-be-your-biggest-meal/

SELFNutritionData, Nutrient data for food listings was provided in part by USDA
Retrieved from http://nutritiondata.self.com/facts/vegetables-and-vegetable-products/2356/2#ixzz4FTlUFOC1

Idea, I. (2014) Meditation 101: Techniques, benefits, and beginners' how-to. Retrieved from http://life.gaiam.com/article/meditation-101-techniques-benefits-beginner-s-how

Cann, K. The science and substance behind your emotional eating. Retrieved from http://breakingmuscle.com/nutrition/the-science-and-substance-behind-your-emotional-eating

Dyer, W. (2012) I Am: Wishes fulfilled meditation. http://www.hayhouse.com/i-am-wishes-fulfilled-meditation

To learn more about or to purchase The 20-Day Full Body Detox visit: **www.lifeandlightwellness.com**

www.ingramcontent.com/pod-product-compliance
Lightning Source LLC
Chambersburg PA
CBHW060908280326
41934CB00007B/1232